Tapping into Herbal Antiviral Powers

Blending Tradition and Science in Fighting Viruses

Emily Watson

Table of Contents

INTRODUCTION 7

CHAPTER I. Understanding Viruses 8

What Are Viruses? 8

The Mechanics of Viral Infections 10

Common Types of Viral Infections 12

CHAPTER II. Herbal Medicine an Overview 16

History and Evolution of Herbal Medicine 16

Key Concepts and Principles.................................... 20

Herbal Medicine's Place in Contemporary Healthcare . 22

CHAPTER III. Traditional Herbal Antivirals 26

Ancient Wisdom: Traditional Herbal Remedies 26

Case Studies: Traditional Herbal Antiviral Practices from Different Cultures 29

The Importance of Tradition in Herbal Medicine 33

CHAPTER IV. Science Behind Herbal Antivirals 36

Exploring the Chemical Composition of Medicinal Plants 36

Research on Herbal Antiviral Efficacy 39

Challenges and Limitations of Herbal Medicine Research 42

CHAPTER V. Common Herbal Antivirals 45

Overview of Key Herbal Antivirals 45

Properties and Mechanisms of Action 49

Usage and Dosage Guidelines 52

CHAPTER VI. Integrating Herbal and Conventional Medicine 56

Understanding the Synergy Between Herbal and Conventional Treatments 56

Collaboration Between Herbalists and Modern Healthcare Practitioners 59

Case Studies: Successful Integrative Approaches 62

CHAPTER VII. Herbal Antivirals in Practice 65

Building Your Herbal Antiviral Toolkit 65

Practical Tips for Incorporating Herbal Remedies into Daily Life 68

Recipes and Formulations for Herbal Antiviral Preparations 71

CHAPTER VIII. Safety and Regulation 75

Ensuring Safety in Herbal Medicine Use 75

Regulatory Framework for Herbal Products 78

Responsible Herbal Medicine Practices 81

CHAPTER IX. Future Directions in Herbal Antiviral Research and Practice 84

Emerging Trends and Innovations 84

Potential Challenges and Opportunities 87

The Role of Herbal Medicine in Global Health Preparedness 91

CHAPTER X. Herbal Medicine in Public Health Initiatives 95

Utilizing Herbal Medicine in Disease Prevention

Campaigns 95

Herbal Medicine in Epidemic and Pandemic Response

Strategies 97

Community-Based Herbal Medicine Programs for

Underserved Populations 100

CHAPTER XI. Ethical Considerations and Cultural

Competence in Herbal Medicine 103

Practice Respecting Cultural Traditions and Indigenous

Knowledge 103

Addressing Ethical Dilemmas in Herbal Medicine

Research and Practice 105

Promoting Cultural Competence and Diversity in Herbal

Medicine Education 108

CHAPTER XII. Herbal Medicine and Mental Health 112

Herbal Remedies for Stress Reduction and Mental Well-

Being 112

Herbal Approaches to Anxiety and Depression

Management 115

Integration of Herbal Medicine into Holistic Mental

Health Care 118

CHAPTER XIII. Herbal Medicine and Chronic Disease

Management 122

Herbal Therapies for Chronic Conditions such as

Diabetes, Hypertension, and Autoimmune Disorders . 122

Herbal Medicine in Integrative Cancer Care 125

Addressing Chronic Pain with Herbal Remedies 127

CHAPTER XIV. Herbal Medicine and Environmental Sustainability **132**

Promoting Sustainable Cultivation and Harvesting Practices 132

Conservation Efforts for Endangered Medicinal Plants 136

CONCLUSION **140**

INTRODUCTION

The ground-breaking study "Tapping into Herbal Antiviral Powers: Blending Tradition and Science in Fighting Viruses" examines how contemporary scientific discoveries and conventional herbal medicines interact to fight viral infections. This book provides a comprehensive strategy incorporating state-of-the-art research and centuries-old wisdom to address viruses' risks to world health.

This book's primary goal is to highlight the beneficial nature of traditional herbal therapy and mainstream healthcare procedures, bridging the gap between them. As they explore the newest scientific findings about the antiviral qualities of medicinal plants, readers will also receive insight into ancient practices from various cultures across the extensive history of herbal medicine.

This book offers helpful advice for integrating herbal medicines into daily life and demystifies herbal therapy through scientific explanations, historical stories, and case studies. Readers will gain the information and skills necessary to successfully traverse the complicated field of viral health, from comprehending the mechanics underlying viral illnesses to investigating the effectiveness and safety of herbal antivirals.

"Tapping into Herbal Antiviral Powers" is more than simply a book; it's a manifesto for utilizing nature's healing powers to combat viruses, giving people looking for natural solutions to safeguard their well-being, health, hope, and empowerment.

CHAPTER I

Understanding Viruses

What Are Viruses?

Viruses are mysterious objects that exist in the gray area between living and non-living materials. Their distinct biology fascinates scientists while also posing severe threats to human health. Viruses are microscopic pathogenic entities consisting of genetic material, either DNA or RNA, encased in a capsid, a protein covering. Viruses, in contrast to bacteria, cannot reproduce on their own; instead, they must subvert the host cell's metabolic functions to multiply.

The astounding diversity of viruses—many species exist in almost every environment on Earth—is one of their most notable characteristics. From simple colds to more dangerous infections like HIV and Ebola, viruses can take many different shapes and sizes and possess distinct characteristics and behaviors. Even though viruses are small, they can have a significant impact on their hosts, causing a variety of illnesses that vary from minor discomfort to severe sickness.

The clever flexibility of viruses is demonstrated by the way they infect host cells. Viruses bind to specific cell surface receptors when they come across a susceptible host and inject their genetic material into the host cell. Once inside, the viral genome seizes control of the cellular apparatus and uses host resources to reproduce its genetic material and make viral proteins. This process frequently leads to cell malfunction or death, exacerbating viral infection symptoms.

The capacity of viruses to quickly adapt to selection forces, such as alterations in host immunity or environmental factors, is one of their most remarkable characteristics. The formation of novel virus strains and the advent of drug-resistant variations demonstrate this evolutionary adaptability and present significant obstacles to medical therapy. Furthermore, viruses are capable of genetic reassortment and recombination, which can develop novel strains with unanticipated characteristics.

Viruses are vital components of ecosystems and biological processes, even though they have the capacity to be harmful. For example, viruses can affect the cycle of nutrients in marine settings by interacting with phytoplankton and bacteria. Additionally, they act as carriers of horizontal gene transfer, which promotes genetic variety by allowing the transfer of genetic material across other organisms.

Viral infections in the context of human health offer both challenges and opportunities. Viral infections have accelerated medical research and technological breakthroughs despite the fact that viruses can cause widespread illness and fatality. The study of viruses has resulted in the creation of diagnostic instruments, antiviral medications, and vaccines that have transformed healthcare and saved countless lives. Moreover, viruses are essential model organisms for studying fundamental biological processes such as evolution, gene expression, and reproduction.

The advent of new viral diseases, including SARS-CoV-2, in recent years, has highlighted the significance of comprehending viruses and creating efficient preventative and therapeutic measures. Given this, herbal therapy offers a potentially effective way to treat viral infections by utilizing the inherent antiviral qualities of medicinal plants to boost immunity and prevent the spread of viruses. By utilizing the extensive history of herbal medicines and fusing them with contemporary scientific understanding, we may fully utilize nature's pharmacy in the continuous fight against viruses.

The Mechanics of Viral Infections

The mechanisms of viral infections result from a convoluted interaction between the virus and its host, involving a sequence of complex molecular processes that lead to the creation and spread of infection. Comprehending these pathways is essential for formulating efficacious antiviral tactics, such as employing herbal treatments to impede virus reproduction and dissemination.

The first stage of a viral infection is when the virus attaches itself to specific receptors on the surface of host cells. To make this first interaction easier, viral surface proteins identify and attach to matching receptor molecules on the surface of host cells. Which cell types the virus can infect is determined by its tropism or target cell specificity, which is determined by the specificity of this interaction. To facilitate viral entrance, the SARS-CoV-2 virus, for instance, attaches to the angiotensin-converting enzyme 2 (ACE2) receptor on human cells through its spike protein.

The process by which the virus enters the host cell after attachment is referred to as viral entrance or penetration. This could occur in a few different ways: the process of directly fusing the viral envelope with the host cell membrane, receptor-mediated endocytosis, or endocytosis. After entering the host cell, the virus needs to find its way around the cellular environment to get to the equipment required for replication. Uncoating is the process of removing the viral capsid to reveal the genetic material of a virus in certain situations.

Now that the viral genome has been revealed, viral replication can start. The virus's replication may occur in the cytoplasm, nucleus, or both of the host cells, depending on the kind and genetic makeup of the virus. DNA viruses usually reproduce inside the nucleus, transcribing viral genes and duplicating viral DNA using the host cell's DNA polymerase and other biological machinery. Conversely, RNA viruses use the viral RNA polymerases encoded in their genomes to reproduce in the cytoplasm.

Viral protein synthesis, viral particle assembly, and viral genome packaging into offspring virions are all part of the highly regulated replication process. Viral proteins perform various functions in this process, such as modulating host cell activity, acting as structural elements of the viral particle, and acting as enzymes for genome replication. New viral particles are frequently assembled at specific locations within the host cell, where viral proteins and nucleic acids are combined to produce mature virions.

Newly created virions must leave the host cell after assembly to infect other cells and spread the infection. Viral egress is the process that results from a variety of mechanisms, such as cell lysis, exocytosis, or budding from the host cell membrane. During their exit, certain viruses pick up an envelope made of the host cell membrane, which can help them avoid the host immune system and spread more easily following infection cycles.

Viruses interact with different parts of the host immune system during an infection, triggering an immunological response that can either control or worsen the infection. The initial line of defense against viral infections is the synthesis of interferons and activating natural killer cells by innate immune systems. Furthermore, generating virus-specific antibodies and cytotoxic T cells are examples of adaptive immune responses vital for eliminating the infection and establishing long-term immunity.

Targeting critical viral life cycle stages in the context of herbal antiviral therapy is a viable strategy for preventing viral replication and dissemination. Numerous antiviral properties of herbal treatments have been demonstrated, including the ability to block viral attachment, entrance, reproduction, and assembly. Herbal antivirals work by interfering with vital stages of the viral life cycle, which can lower the viral load, treat symptoms, and strengthen the host immune system.

In summary, complex molecular processes that determine the course of infection control the mechanics of viral infections. Viral methods range from attachment and entry to replication, assembly, and egress, all aimed at taking advantage of host cells and spreading infection. Comprehending these pathways is crucial for creating effective antiviral treatments, such as using herbal remedies to treat viral infections. Herbal antivirals provide a potentially effective way to improve our capacity to manage and treat viral diseases by explicitly targeting essential stages of the viral life cycle.

Common Types of Viral Infections

Frequent viral infections are associated with a wide range of illnesses that affect people worldwide, from minor respiratory conditions to severe and often fatal conditions. Numerous viruses from various families, each with distinct traits and clinical signs, are the source of these diseases. It is imperative to understand the common forms of viral infections to effectively prevent, diagnose, and treat viral infections, including herbal antiviral medicines to boost the body's immune response and inhibit viral reproduction.

Each year, millions of people are afflicted with respiratory viral infections, which are among the most common viral disorders. Cough, fever, nasal congestion, and sore throat are common symptoms of respiratory viruses, which include influenza viruses, respiratory syncytial virus (RSV), and coronaviruses. These viruses usually target the respiratory system. In particular, influenza is recognized for its capacity to trigger sporadic pandemics and seasonal epidemics, which significantly increase global morbidity and mortality rates. Similar to this, coronaviruses have become significant threats to public health in recent years, causing widespread illness and global economic disruption. Examples of these include the Middle East respiratory syndrome coronavirus (MERS- CoV), the novel coronavirus SARS-CoV-2 that is responsible for COVID-19, and the severe acute respiratory syndrome coronavirus (SARS-CoV).

Gastroenteritis is another common viral infection affecting the gastrointestinal tract and causes symptoms like fever, diarrhea, vomiting, and abdominal pain. In environments like schools, daycare centers, and hospitals, intestinal viruses—such as norovirus, rotavirus, and adenovirus— can spread quickly and are highly contagious. While most viral gastroenteritis cases are self-limiting and go away in a few days, severe instances can result in electrolyte imbalances and dehydration, especially in small children, older people, and people with impaired immune systems.

Another important class of viral infections that affects the liver and, if ignored, can result in cirrhosis, hepatocellular carcinoma, and chronic liver disease is viral hepatitis. Different varieties of hepatitis viruses are recognized, such as hepatitis A, B, C, D, and also E. Each variety has a unique clinical course, transmission mechanism, and treatment. Bloodborne pathways, including intravenous drug use, sexual contact, and perinatal transmission, mainly disseminate Hepatitis B, C, and D. Hepatitis A and E are usually spread by contaminated food and water. For some forms of viral hepatitis, there are antiviral medications and vaccinations against hepatitis viruses, although access to these treatments is still restricted in many regions of the world.

Due to their ubiquity, chronic nature, and potential for long-term problems, sexually transmitted viruses like the human papillomavirus (HPV), herpes simplex virus (HSV), and human immunodeficiency virus (HIV) provide public severe health challenges. That being said, HPV is the most common STD worldwide, with over 100 different genotypes. Some of these genotypes have been linked to oropharyngeal, cervical, and anal malignancies as well as genital warts. Recurrent oral and vaginal sores are caused by HSV, which is comprised of herpes simplex virus types 1 (HSV-1) and 2 (HSV-2). HSV can be spread by close personal contact or sexual interaction. Acquired immunodeficiency syndrome (AIDS), which exacerbates immunosuppression and increases a person's susceptibility to cancer and opportunistic infections, is brought on by the HIV virus, which targets the immune system. Despite advances in antiretroviral medication, HIV/AIDS remains a primary worldwide health concern, particularly in underdeveloped countries where access to treatment and preventative measures is restricted.

Apart from these prevalent forms of viral infections, many different viral ailments can impact diverse organ systems and tissues across the body. Hemorrhagic fevers, meningitis, viral encephalitis, and myocarditis are a few examples, each of which poses particular difficulties in diagnosis, care, and prevention. Furthermore, there is a constant need for surveillance, study, and preparation since viral infections, including the Zika, chikungunya, and Ebola viruses, continue to pose unanticipated dangers to the security of global health.

Targeting common viral infections in the context of herbal antiviral therapy necessitates a multimodal strategy that considers each virus's unique traits and mechanisms. Since ancient times, people have utilized herbal treatments to treat viral infections. These medicines enhance the body's innate immune response, prevent viral replication, and reduce symptoms. Through knowledge of common viral infections and how they cause illness, researchers and medical professionals can find promising herbal antiviral agents and create evidence- based treatment plans that provide safe, efficient, and cost-effective substitutes for traditional therapies.

CHAPTER II

Herbal Medicine an Overview

History and Evolution of Herbal Medicine

Herbal medicine has a long history that begins at the birth of human civilization, long before written records existed when plants were used for therapeutic purposes. Ancient civilizations, including the Egyptians, Greeks, Chinese, and Indigenous peoples of the Americas, relied on herbs' medicinal qualities to treat various illnesses and enhance overall health and well-being. These practices were practiced throughout nations and continents. Through trial and error, these early healers learned about the effects of herbs on the human body and verbally transmitted their knowledge from generation to generation.

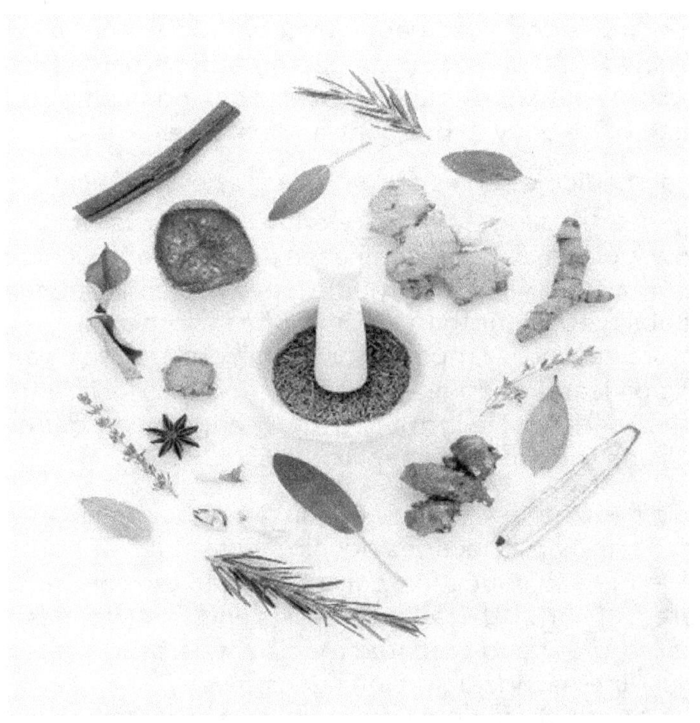

Medicinal plants were essential to embalming procedures, healthcare, and religious rites in ancient Egypt. The Ebers Papyrus, which dates to circa 1550 BCE, showcases the advanced knowledge of herbal medicine in ancient Egyptian civilization by providing in-depth descriptions of hundreds of medicinal plants and their therapeutic applications. Comparably, prominent Greek authors like Hippocrates and Dioscorides recorded the therapeutic qualities of plants in their works, establishing the groundwork for modern Western herbal therapy.

Traditional Chinese medicine (TCM), which has been practiced for more than 2,000 years, views herbs, acupuncture, massage, and food therapy as vital components of holistic healing. Thousands of medical substances, such as herbs, minerals, and animal products, are included in the Chinese materia medica. These compounds are categorized based on their flavor, temperature, and therapeutic effects. Traditional Chinese medicine (TCM) practitioners recommend herbal formulas based on a patient's unique constitution and health issues to restore the body to harmony and balance.

Herbal medicine serves as the mainstay of healthcare in indigenous healing traditions worldwide. For example, yarrow, goldenseal, and echinacea are among the herbs used by Native American medicine women and men for their ability to strengthen the immune system and promote healing. Comparably, through oral traditions and hands-on learning, traditional healers in Africa, Asia, and South America have ingrained knowledge of indigenous plants and their medical applications.

During the Middle Ages and Renaissance, botanical gardens and apothecaries developed as hubs of herbal knowledge and education, contributing to the continuous progress of herbal therapy. Herbalists and apothecaries gathered, grew, and prepared medicinal herbs to treat various illnesses, including infections, fevers, gastrointestinal problems, and skin issues. Herbal knowledge was further disseminated, and herbal medicines were standardized to produce herbals and illustrated manuals detailing medicinal plants and their uses.

Herbal medicine saw a fall in popularity as pharmaceuticals and technological advancements replaced traditional medical practices with the rise of modern medicine in the 19th and 20th centuries. But in recent decades, there has been a rebirth of interest in natural and holistic remedies, which has led to a renewed understanding of herbs' medicinal properties. Herbal medicine's rise as a supplementary and alternative medical practice has been fueled by scientific studies into the pharmacological characteristics of medicinal plants, which have confirmed numerous ancient uses and shown new therapeutic applications.

Herbal medicine is becoming widely accepted and popular as more people look for sustainable and natural ways to improve their health and well-being. To meet the increasing demand for plant-based medications, herbal supplements, teas, tinctures, and topical therapies are easily accessible in pharmacies, health food stores, and internet merchants. Furthermore, as medical professionals understand the importance of treating the underlying causes of disease and fostering whole-body recovery, integrative healthcare approaches—which mix traditional medicine with herbal and holistic therapies— are spreading more widely.

Herbal medicine provides a multitude of potential solutions for fighting viral infections when used in conjunction with antiviral treatment. Numerous herbs have antiviral qualities that can reduce the growth of viruses, alter the immune system, and lessen the symptoms of viral infections. For ages, people have utilized herbal remedies, including echinacea, elderberry, licorice root, and astragalus, to cure and prevent viral infections. Current research has shown these remedies' effectiveness in enhancing immune system performance and mitigating the intensity and length of symptoms.

The development and history of herbal medicine offer essential insights into the therapeutic value of plants and the long-standing bond between people and the natural environment. Through the integration of contemporary scientific understanding with this age-old wisdom, we may effectively utilize the medicinal properties of herbs to enhance well-being, fend off illness, and battle viral infections. Using herbal remedies to combat viruses that threaten human health and well-being is a combination of science and tradition that offers hope and healing.

Key Concepts and Principles

The fundamental ideas and precepts of herbal medicine guide the application and practice of this age-old therapeutic modality. These ideas, which have their roots in conventional knowledge and are bolstered by current scientific studies, offer a framework for comprehending the therapeutic qualities of medicinal plants and their function in enhancing health and well-being.

The idea of holism, which sees the body as a complex and interrelated system with physical, mental, emotional, and spiritual qualities, is one of the core ideas of herbal medicine. From this angle, health is a condition of harmony and balance in the body and mind rather than only the absence of sickness. Rather than focusing only on treating symptoms, herbalists work to address the underlying causes of sickness and bring the body's systems back into balance.

The idea of individualization, which acknowledges that every person is different and may react differently to herbal therapies depending on aspects including constitution, heredity, lifestyle, and environment, is another fundamental tenet of herbal therapy. Herbalists approach healthcare with a tailored approach, creating treatment programs specific to each patient while considering their preferences, medical history, and general state of health. The choice and application of herbal treatments can be made with more freedom and personalization thanks to this tailored method.

Additionally, herbal medicine emphasizes the value of proactive healthcare and prevention above the reactive treatment provided after an ailment has already developed. Herbal treatments can assist in preventing disease and improve resilience to environmental stresses and infections by bolstering the body's natural defenses and innate healing systems. The goals of holistic medicine, which emphasize the preservation of health and vitality through dietary changes, stress reduction methods, and lifestyle adjustments, align with this preventive approach to health.

The idea of vitalism, which holds that all living things have an innate life force or vital energy that controls their growth, development, and health, is fundamental to herbal medicine. Herbalists contend that this life-giving force is present in medicinal plants in bioactive chemicals that, when applied topically or consumed internally, have therapeutic effects on the body. Herbalists use plants' therapeutic properties to help rebalance and energize the body's life energy, which promotes resilience and overall health.

The significance of ecological care and sustainability in gathering, growing, and preserving therapeutic plants is also emphasized by herbal medicine. A large number of therapeutic plants come from wild populations that are at risk from habitat degradation, overharvesting, and climate change. Herbalists support ethical wildcrafting techniques, conscientious cultivation methods, and the preservation of endangered species to guarantee the long-term availability of therapeutic plants and maintain biodiversity. Furthermore, organic farming, agroforestry, and permaculture are being promoted as sustainable alternatives to conventional agriculture—which primarily relies on chemical inputs and monoculture and cropping systems.

The pharmacological characteristics and methods of action of medicinal plants have been better understood in recent years thanks to scientific research, which has also provided important insights into these plants' safety and therapeutic potential. Herbalists use this evidence-based knowledge to guide the selection of suitable herbs for specific health issues and to inform their practice. However, it's critical to understand that herbal medicine is a science and an art and that empirical observations and traditional knowledge are just as significant in directing herbal practice.

The selection, preparation, and administration of herbal remedies for treating viral infections are guided by fundamental concepts and principles of herbal medicine in the context of antiviral therapy. When creating treatment plans, herbalists consider variables, including the virus's aggressiveness, the patient's constitution, and the infection's stage. To combat the virus, boost immunity, and lessen symptoms related to viral infections, they might use a blend of herbs having antiviral, immune-stimulating, and anti-inflammatory qualities.

In summary, fundamental ideas and precepts serve as the cornerstone of herbal medicine, directing practitioners to advance well-being, fend off illness, and reestablish mental and physical equilibrium. Herbalists use the therapeutic power of plants to promote people's health and well-being while adhering to the principles of sustainability, vitalism, individualization, preventative, and evidence-based practice.

Leveraging the antiviral properties of herbs is a blend of conventional knowledge and contemporary research, providing comfort and restoration when confronted with viral dangers to human well-being.

Herbal Medicine's Place in Contemporary Healthcare

Herbal medicine plays a diverse role in contemporary healthcare, with applications ranging from evidence-based treatments and integrative approaches to health and wellness to traditional folk remedies. Phytotherapy, botanical medicine, and herbal medicine are terms used to describe the medical application of plants and plant-derived substances to cure, prevent, or treat a range of ailments. Herbal therapy has been used in many societies and cultures for thousands of years. Still, its comeback in contemporary medicine results from a growing understanding of the therapeutic value of medicinal plants and the drawbacks of traditional pharmaceutical therapies.

Herbal medicine is a complementary and alternative therapy for controlling chronic health issues and enhancing general well-being, one of its primary functions in contemporary healthcare. For illnesses like arthritis, diabetes, cardiovascular disease, and gastrointestinal issues, many people use herbal remedies as an adjuvant to traditional medications. Herbal remedies promote the body's natural healing processes and address the underlying causes of sickness, providing a natural and comprehensive approach to healthcare. Herbal medicines are also often less likely to cause adverse effects and drug interactions than pharmaceutical treatments, which makes them suitable for long-term use and integration into customized treatment regimens.

Herbal medications are essential for addressing chronic illnesses, but they also promote organ health, lower inflammation, and boost immunological function, all of which are essential aspects of preventative healthcare. Supplements containing herbal ingredients like echinacea, elderberry, and astragalus are frequently used to support the body's defenses against viral infections, which include respiratory tract infections, influenza, and the common cold. Popular preventive treatments include herbal teas, tinctures, and tonics, which offer a fun and straightforward approach to including medicinal plants in everyday activities.

Many people realize that herbal therapy is an effective way to address acute health issues, such as minor wounds, infections, and digestive issues. A rising number of people searching for natural alternatives to conventional over-the-counter medications are turning to herbal first aid packs filled with remedies like calendula for burns and wounds, arnica for sprains and bruises, and ginger for nausea and dyspepsia. Herbal treatments have the potential to accelerate healing and offer quick symptom relief without the adverse side effects that come with some pharmaceutical medications.

Herbal medicine plays a significant part in creating new drugs and modern healthcare. Plants, fungi, and microbes are among the natural sources of many pharmaceutical medications. Herbal medicine offers a wealth of bioactive chemicals that may have therapeutic uses. Investigations into the pharmacological characteristics of therapeutic plants have produced new compounds with antibacterial, antiviral, anti-inflammatory, and anticancer properties, among other effects. These findings could lead to the creation of novel medications and treatment approaches for a variety of illnesses.

Additionally, the promotion of ecological stewardship and environmental sustainability in healthcare is greatly aided by herbal medicine. Herbal medications are obtained from renewable plant sources and cultivated using sustainable agricultural practices, unlike traditional pharmaceutical treatments, which are often created from synthetic chemicals and produced using ecologically destructive processes. For those who are worried about the environmental impact of their healthcare decisions, herbal therapies are a more environmentally friendly option because they are often biodegradable and have a low ecological impact.

Patients and healthcare professionals are beginning to favor integrative healthcare methods that blend traditional medicine with complementary and alternative therapies, including herbal and holistic remedies. Integrative medicine combines the best aspects of traditional and complementary medicine to offer complete and individualized care, acknowledging the importance of promoting health and recovery. Integrative healthcare techniques heavily rely on herbal medicine, which provides a natural, all-encompassing approach to health that enhances traditional medical interventions.

Herbal medicine provides many potential treatments for fighting viral infections and bolstering immune function when used with antiviral therapy. Numerous therapeutic plants have antiviral qualities that can reduce the growth of viruses, alter the immune system, and lessen the symptoms of viral infections. An effective way to strengthen the body's defenses against viral infections and aid in healing is through integrative approaches to antiviral therapy, which blends traditional medical interventions with herbal therapies.

In summary, herbal medicine plays various roles in contemporary healthcare and is continuously developing to meet the demands of the changing healthcare landscape. Herbal medicine offers a comprehensive approach to health and healing based on tradition, backed by science, and accepted by people and communities worldwide. It covers various topics, from drug development and ecological sustainability to preventative healthcare and managing chronic diseases. In the face of viral threats to human health and resilience, harnessing the antiviral properties of herbs is a synthesis of traditional knowledge and contemporary understanding, providing hope and healing.

CHAPTER III

Traditional Herbal Antivirals

Ancient Wisdom: Traditional Herbal Remedies

Traditional herbal treatments and ancient wisdom are intricately entwined, representing both the long-lasting human-plant interaction and the complex tapestry of human experience. Ancient healers from all nations and civilizations depended on the therapeutic properties of medicinal plants to prevent, treat, and mitigate various illnesses, including viral infections. Traditional herbal remedies, which have their roots in centuries-old customs and have been handed down through the generations, represent the collective knowledge of our predecessors and provide essential insights into the medicinal potential of plants.

Medicinal herbs were the primary healthcare source for most people worldwide in the past, long before pharmaceutical pharmaceuticals became widely available. Native American, Aboriginal Australian, and African tribal civilizations, among others, profoundly understand the therapeutic qualities of nearby plants and employ them to enhance their well-being. Oral tradition, experimentation, and observation were the foundation for these ancient therapeutic systems. Elders imparted their knowledge of herbs to younger generations through storytelling and apprenticeship.

Traditional herbal medicines are known for their holistic approach to healing, which acknowledges the connection between the mind, body, and spirit. Traditional healers recognized that being healthy encompasses more than just being free from illness; it also involves a person's environment and internal balance. In addition to treating specific symptoms, herbal treatments were recommended to address fundamental imbalances and help the body return to its normal equilibrium. Many traditional treatment systems, such as Ayurveda, traditional Chinese medicine, and Indigenous healing traditions, still strongly emphasize this holistic approach.

Because traditional herbal cures are frequently made from plants that are easily found and abundant in the surrounding area, even populations with little resources can afford and use them. Expert botanists and herbalists with in-depth knowledge of the indigenous flora's medicinal applications made up many traditional healers. They knew which plants to gather, when and how to do so, and how to prepare and use them for the most therapeutic benefit. Ancient healers could sustainably and environmentally friendlyly utilize the therapeutic power of plants because of their close relationship with the natural world.

Traditional herbal medicines have been used for a long time to cure various illnesses, including viral infections. Since ancient times, people have employed plants with immune-stimulating and antiviral qualities, such as licorice, echinacea, elderberry, garlic, and ginger, to prevent and treat respiratory infections, including colds and the flu. In addition to food and lifestyle suggestions to promote general health and immunity, these cures were frequently given as teas, tinctures, poultices, and salves.

Apart from their immediate medicinal benefits, ancient herbal treatments frequently held a pivotal position in cultural and spiritual customs, functioning as emblems of recovery, safeguarding, and association with the natural world. In their healing rituals, many Indigenous nations considered certain plants sacred companions and sought advice from plant spirits and deities. Invoking divine blessings and healing energies, herbal medicines were frequently accompanied by prayers, chants, and ceremonies. These practices gave herbal treatments a symbolic meaning and significance.

Traditional herbal medicines are still widely used worldwide despite the advances in modern medicine. This is particularly true in impoverished and rural places where there is little access to conventional medical care. Known by various titles, including herbalists, medicine men, and shamans, traditional healers are essential to maintaining cultural traditions and offering healthcare services. They are regarded as a great benefit to society and frequently pass down their knowledge of native plants and their medical uses orally.

Growing knowledge of pharmaceutical medications' drawbacks and adverse effects has led to a renaissance of interest in traditional herbal therapies among mainstream consumers and healthcare professionals in recent years. As a more natural and safe alternative to traditional medical care, herbal therapy is gaining popularity. This is especially true for chronic illnesses and symptoms associated with specific lifestyle choices. Many health food stores, pharmacies, and internet vendors carry herbal supplements, teas, and topical therapies that address various health issues.

Traditional herbal medicines provide many choices for fighting viral infections and bolstering immune function when used with antiviral therapy. For ages, traditional medical systems worldwide have employed plants like elderberry, licorice root, astragalus, and olive leaf to prevent and treat viral infections. These herbs are essential partners in the fight against viral infections because they contain bioactive substances with antiviral, immune-stimulating, and anti-inflammatory activities.

In conclusion, traditional herbal treatments and age-old wisdom offer a therapeutic legacy ending in the present era. Traditional herbal remedies, which have their roots in centuries-old customs and have been handed down through the generations, provide essential insights into the medicinal potential of plants and their function in enhancing health and well-being. The full potential of herbal medicine to sustain our health and vitality in the face of viral threats and other health difficulties can be realized by honoring our ancestors' wisdom and harnessing plants' healing power.

Case Studies: Traditional Herbal Antiviral Practices from Different Cultures

Case studies of traditional herbal antiviral techniques from numerous societies illustrate the rich tapestry of human experience in fighting viral infections and provide insightful information on the various approaches to plant-based therapy. Traditional healers have created distinctive herbal cures and treatment plans based on regional plant resources, cultural values, and indigenous knowledge across continents and civilizations. These case reports demonstrate the continued effectiveness of herbal therapy and offer guidance for future research and clinical applications.

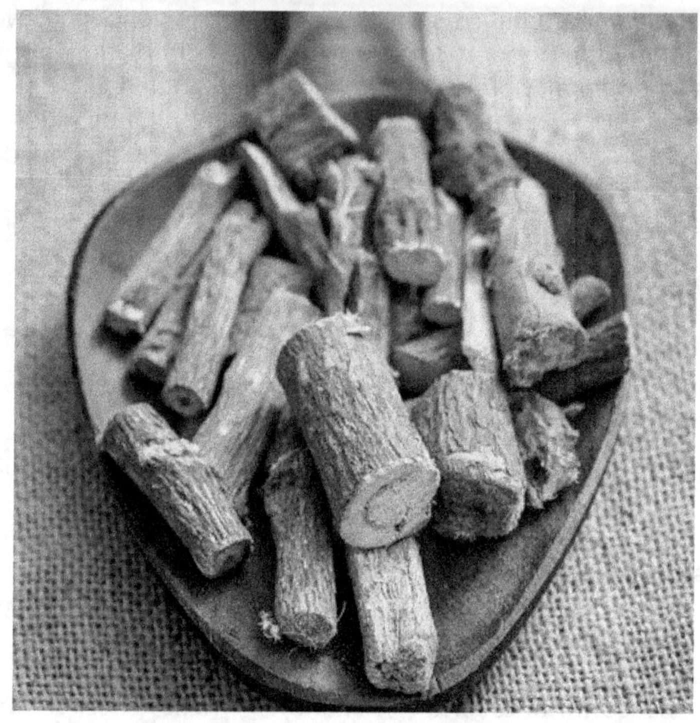

Traditional Chinese medicine (TCM) has long employed herbs, such as astragalus (Huang Qi), licorice root (Gan Cao), and honeysuckle flower (Jin Yin Hua), to prevent and treat viral infections. Astragalus is often used as a tonic herb to enhance general vitality and strengthen the body's defenses because of its immune-stimulating properties. Licorice root removes heat and toxins from the body and relieves respiratory infection symptoms because of its antiviral and anti-inflammatory properties. The blossom honeysuckle is highly valued for its capacity to eliminate lung heat and toxins. It is frequently applied as a remedy for fever, sore throats, and other symptoms associated with viral respiratory diseases. Yin Qiao San and Yu Ping Feng San are two standard traditional formulae that combine these herbs to maximize their synergistic effects and treat the underlying imbalances brought on by viral infections.

Herbs like tulsi (Ocimum sanctum), Curcuma longa (Curcuma longa), and neem (Azadirachta indica) are valued for their antiviral qualities in Ayurvedic medicine, the ancient Indian healing system. Respected for its broad-spectrum antibacterial activity, neem is sometimes called the "village pharmacy" in India. It is used to treat various infectious disorders, including viral infections. Tulsi, or holy basil, is highly valued in Ayurveda for its immune-boosting and antiviral qualities. Due to its powerful antiviral and anti-inflammatory qualities, curcumin, the main ingredient in turmeric, is frequently used to boost immunity and lessen inflammation caused by viral infections. These plants enhance health and lifespan in classic Ayurvedic formulations like Triphala and Chyawanprash.

Plants such as osha root (Ligusticum porteri), elderberry (Sambucus nigra), and echinacea (Echinacea purpurea) have been utilized for generations in Native American medicinal practices to prevent and treat viral infections. Purple coneflower, or echinacea, is highly valued for its immune-stimulating qualities and is used to ward off respiratory diseases such as the flu and colds.

Elderberries are prized for their antiviral and immune-boosting properties and are frequently used to treat influenza and other viral infections because of their high flavonoid and anthocyanin content. Osha root is used in traditional medicine to treat respiratory illnesses like pneumonia, the flu, and colds. It is prized for its antibacterial and immune-modulating qualities and is utilized by Native American tribes living in the Rocky Mountains. These herbs are used topically or orally to treat viral diseases and reduce symptoms. They are frequently made into teas, tinctures, or syrups.

African traditional medicine uses herbs, including Sutherlandia (Sutherlandia frutescens), African potato (Hypoxis hemerocallis), and African ginger (Zingiber officinale), to prevent and treat viral illnesses. African ginger, sometimes called "lemon ginger" or "yellow ginger," is valued for its anti-inflammatory and immune-stimulating qualities and is used to treat respiratory illnesses like the flu and colds. Native to South Africa, the African potato is a tuberous plant prized for its antioxidant and immune-stimulating properties. It treats viral diseases by reducing inflammation and bolstering the immune system. Sutherlandia, commonly referred to as "the cancer bush," is used to treat a range of infectious disorders, such as hepatitis and HIV/AIDS, and is highly regarded for its immune-modulating and antiviral qualities. These herbs are used topically or orally to support health; they are frequently made into tinctures, decoctions, or infusions.

Plants like cat's claw (Uncaria tomentosa), Suma (Pfaffia paniculata), and pau d'arco (Tabebuia impetiginosa) are utilized in indigenous medicine traditions of the Americas to prevent and treat viral infections. Pau d'arco, popularly called "Taheebo" or "Lapacho," is valued for its antiviral, antibacterial, and antifungal characteristics and is utilized in the treatment of numerous infectious disorders, such as herpes, the common cold, and the flu. Cat's claw, so called because of its claw-like thorns, is used to support immune function and reduce inflammation in viral diseases. It is prized for its immuno-modulating and anti-inflammatory properties. Suma, sometimes called "Brazilian ginseng," is prized for its immune-stimulating and adaptogenic qualities and promotes vigor and resilience against illness and stress. These herbs are taken orally to support health and energy; they are frequently made into teas, tinctures, or capsules.

Finally, case studies of traditional herbal antiviral techniques from many cultures demonstrate the variety of plant-based medical approaches and the long-lasting effectiveness of traditional therapeutic systems in the fight against viral infections. by paying tribute to our forefathers' knowledge.

The Importance of Tradition in Herbal Medicine

It is impossible to overestimate the significance of tradition in herbal medicine since it forms the foundation for the field's contemporary application. Through oral tradition, written texts, and cultural practices, many generations of healers have passed down their insights and skills, accumulating a wealth of wisdom, knowledge, and experience collectively called tradition. Within the field of herbal medicine, tradition offers a framework for comprehending the therapeutic qualities of medicinal plants along with the guidelines and customs surrounding their application.

The understanding that plants are essential to human health and well-being is one of the central tenets of the herbal medicine tradition. Plants have been integral to regular medical procedures, spiritual ceremonies, and healing rituals for thousands of years. The fundamental link that exists between humans and the natural world was recognized by traditional healers, who also knew that plants had inherent therapeutic qualities that could be used to enhance health and vitality. By upholding this age-old custom, contemporary herbalists continue to use historical knowledge to direct their work and shape their therapeutic approaches.

The emphasis on holistic health and wellness is crucial to the tradition of herbal medicine. The body, mind, and spirit are interrelated, and traditional healing systems like Ayurveda, traditional Chinese medicine, and Indigenous healing traditions aim to treat the underlying causes of sickness rather than just its symptoms. Herbal treatments are considered a holistic approach to health that includes dietary adjustments, lifestyle interventions, and spiritual activities that are all intended to help the individual regain harmony and balance in their life. Modern herbalists can address health issues with greater efficacy and sustainability by adopting this holistic viewpoint.

Another critical factor in guaranteeing the security and effectiveness of herbal remedies is tradition. Traditional healers have used a great deal of empirical observation and experimentation throughout history to identify the curative qualities of medicinal plants and the right amounts and preparations for them. The foundation of traditional herbal pharmacopeias and materia medicas—which act as archives of herbal wisdom and instruction for practitioners—is this empirical information that has been passed down through the generations. Modern herbalists can guarantee the safety, efficacy, and quality of their prescribed herbal therapies by upholding traditional beliefs and methods.

Traditional herbal medicines provide both medical and spiritual benefits, but they also have cultural and spiritual value for the communities that use them. Sacred allies and many medicinal plants are included in healing rituals, rites of passage, and cultural traditions. To preserve traditional knowledge and practices for future generations, traditional healers function as guardians of this cultural heritage. Modern herbalists can enhance the healing process by cultivating a stronger bond with the plants and the people they serve by respecting the cultural traditions connected to herbal medicine.

In addition, tradition gives people a feeling of resilience and continuity in the face of social, economic, and environmental difficulties. Traditional healers have always modified their methods to fit shifting conditions, bringing in fresh herbs, methods, and perspectives while holding fast to their therapeutic philosophies' essential ideas and ideals. The value of tradition in herbal medicine offers a framework for negotiating uncertainty and adversity in today's world of rapid change, acting as a source of strength and stability. Modern herbalists can ensure herbal medicine's continued relevance and efficacy in the twenty-first century by embracing traditional wisdom and values and developing resilience and adaptability in their profession.

The value of tradition in herbal medicine is evident when considering antiviral medication. For years, people have used and tested traditional herbal medicines for viral infections, handed down through the generations. These treatments frequently combine several herbs that enhance immune system performance, prevent the spread of viruses, and synergistically reduce symptoms. Modern herbalists can access a plethora of information and expertise to guide the development of efficient treatment procedures for viral infections by utilizing traditional antiviral methods from various cultures.

To sum up, the importance of tradition in herbal therapy cannot be overstated. A foundation for comprehending the therapeutic qualities of medicinal plants, as well as the values and customs guiding their application, is provided by tradition. Modern herbalists can guarantee herbal medicine's security, effectiveness, and cultural significance in the twenty-first century by upholding ancient wisdom and values. Combining traditional herbal medicine with contemporary science, herbal antiviral therapies provide hope and healing when viruses threaten human health and resilience.

CHAPTER IV

Science Behind Herbal Antivirals

Exploring the Chemical Composition of Medicinal Plants

Investigating the chemical makeup of medicinal plants reveals the complex molecular architecture and bioactive ingredients that support their therapeutic qualities. Plants have evolved various chemical defenses and secondary metabolites to protect themselves from environmental stressors and diseases, spanning varied environments and botanical species. For ages, traditional herbal therapy has utilized the pharmacological qualities of several phytochemicals that humans have utilized. Researchers can find novel chemicals with potential applications in antiviral therapy and other healthcare domains by exploring the chemical composition of medicinal plants.

Alkaloids are a significant family of bioactive compounds in medicinal plants. These molecules contain nitrogen and have a variety of physiological effects. Alkaloids have been used for millennia to treat a variety of illnesses. Well-known examples of these include quinine, morphine, and caffeine. Alkaloids with antiviral properties against a range of viruses, including herpesviruses, influenza, and HIV, are found in plants such as cinchona, which includes quinine; Ephedra sinica, which contains ephedrine; and Catharanthus roseus, which contains vinblastine and vincristine.

Flavonoids are a significant class of phytochemicals that are present in medicinal plants. They are polyphenolic compounds that have immune-modulating, anti-inflammatory, and antioxidant qualities. Fruits, vegetables, and herbs are rich in flavonoids, like quercetin, kaempferol, and epigallocatechin gallate (EGCG), which have been the subject of much research due to their possible health advantages. Empirical studies indicate that certain flavonoids exhibit antiviral properties through their ability to impede viral reproduction, obstruct viral entry into host cells, and regulate immunological responses. For instance, it has been demonstrated that quercetin, present in onions, apples, and tea, inhibits the growth of viruses, including Zika, hepatitis C, and influenza.

Terpenoids, or isoprenoids, are a broad class of phytochemicals in medicinal plants, including triterpenes, steroids, and essential oils. Terpenoids have a variety of biological properties, such as antiviral, antibacterial, and anti-inflammatory properties. Many essential oils derived from aromatic plants, including tea tree, thyme, and eucalyptus oils, have long been used to treat respiratory virus infections due to their potent antiviral properties. Terpenoids are hypothesized to have antiviral properties because of their capacity to influence host immunological responses, damage viral membranes, and inhibit viral enzymes.

Fruits, vegetables, and medicinal plants are rich in polyphenols, which include tannins and phenolic acids. These compounds have drawn interest due to their possible health-promoting properties. Due to their antiviral, anti-inflammatory, and antioxidant characteristics, polyphenols are excellent choices for antiviral treatment. It has been demonstrated that some compounds, such as tannic acid, which is present in tea and red wine, and ellagic acid, which is present in berries and nuts, can prevent the reproduction of some viruses, including the human papillomavirus (HPV), the herpes simplex virus, and influenza. Additionally, polyphenols can improve antiviral defenses, alter host immunological responses, and lessen viral infection-related inflammation.

Another class of phytochemicals with possible antiviral activity is saponins, also known as steroids or glycosylated triterpenes. The biological effects of saponins are diverse and include immune-stimulating, antibacterial, and anti-inflammatory characteristics. Plants high in saponins, such as ginseng, licorice, and soapwort, are used in many traditional herbal treatments for viral infections. According to research, saponins can prevent the multiplication of viruses by rupturing their membranes, preventing them from entering host cells, and boosting the host's immune system. For instance, it has been demonstrated that the active ingredients in ginseng, called ginsenosides, have antiviral properties against the human immunodeficiency virus (HIV), herpes simplex virus (HSV), and respiratory syncytial virus (RSV).

Medicinal plants also include a wide range of additional bioactive substances with possible antiviral qualities, such as lignans, coumarins, polysaccharides, and peptides, in addition to these prominent families of phytochemicals. Numerous substances work together to achieve their therapeutic goals, influencing host immune responses and focusing on various phases of the viral replication cycle. Researchers can find new directions for drug discovery and development by examining the chemical makeup of medicinal plants. This may result in the development of novel antiviral therapies.

To sum up, investigating the chemical makeup of therapeutic plants uncovers a wealth of bioactive substances that may be used in antiviral treatment. Alkaloids, flavonoids, terpenoids, polyphenols, saponins, and other phytochemicals have a variety of pharmacological characteristics that can reduce the growth of viruses, strengthen the host's immune system, and lessen the symptoms of viral infections. Researchers can create new antiviral medications and treatments to fight new viral threats and enhance world health by utilizing the therapeutic potential of medicinal plants. Utilizing herbal remedies with antiviral properties reflects a synthesis of contemporary science and traditional knowledge, providing comfort and hope in the face of viral dangers to human health and adaptability.

Research on Herbal Antiviral Efficacy

An emerging area of research on the effectiveness of herbal antivirals shows potential for developing new remedies for viral infections. Antiviral medicines are desperately needed as the prevalence of viral infections rises worldwide due to urbanization, climate change, and globalization. These therapies must be safe, efficient, and reasonably priced. Based on millennia of traditional use and empirical observation, herbal medicines provide an abundant source of bioactive chemicals that may have antiviral properties. Researchers can uncover bioactive molecules with antiviral capabilities, clarify the mechanisms of action of herbal treatments, and assess the safety and efficacy of these compounds in preclinical and clinical studies by rigorously scientifically examining medicinal plants.

Using in vitro cell culture models, plant extracts and isolated chemicals are screened for activity against particular viruses to study herbal remedies' antiviral efficiency. Using this preliminary screening procedure, scientists can find potential candidates for more investigation based on their capacity to suppress viral growth, obstruct viral entry into host cells, or alter host immune responses. For instance, scientists have discovered many therapeutic plants that exhibit antiviral solid properties against coronaviruses, including SARS-CoV-2, influenza, and respiratory syncytial virus (RSV). Researchers can find fresh possibilities for developing antiviral drugs by screening various plant species.

Using molecular and cellular biology methods, researchers can examine the mechanisms of action of putative antiviral drugs once they have been identified. This entails identifying the precise molecular targets and pathways that herbal remedies use to carry out their antiviral actions, such as modifying host immunological signaling pathways, inhibiting viral replication enzymes, or preventing viral attachment proteins. To maximize the therapeutic efficiency of herbal antiviral compounds, reduce the possibility of side effects, and find synergistic interactions with conventional antiviral medications, it is essential to understand the mechanisms of action of these compounds.

Preclinical research with animal models provides essential information on the safety and effectiveness of herbal antiviral treatments in vivo. Researchers can evaluate herbal treatments' pharmacokinetics, biodistribution, and toxicity and their capacity to stop or lessen viral pathogenesis and transmission using animal models of viral infection, such as mice, ferrets, and non-human primates. These investigations offer vital preclinical information to assist in creating herbal antiviral medications and to guide the planning of human subjects' clinical trials.

Clinical research is the gold standard for assessing the efficacy and safety of herbal antiviral treatments for people. In patients with viral infections, randomized controlled trials (RCTs) are used to evaluate the therapeutic benefits of herbal therapies compared to placebo or standard care therapy. Reduction of the viral load, symptom alleviation, illness progression, and death rates are examples of clinical endpoints. Through a thorough assessment of herbal antiviral treatments in carefully planned clinical studies, scientists can produce strong proof of their safety, effectiveness, and application in medical practice.

Researchers are assessing the effectiveness of herbal antiviral treatments and looking at potential drug-drug interactions and resistance mechanisms. Resistance to antiviral medications is a severe worry in the study of virology. There is mounting evidence, however, that suggests herbal medicines may selectively influence viral populations, creating resistant forms of the virus. To reduce the danger of resistance and extend the effectiveness of antiviral treatments, it is essential to comprehend the mechanisms underlying viral resistance to herbal antiviral agents.

Additionally, herbal remedies may interact with other pharmaceuticals, including conventional antiviral treatments, in ways that could have unanticipated pharmacokinetic and pharmacodynamic effects. Therapeutic-herb interactions can affect therapeutic efficacy or raise the risk of side effects at different levels, including absorption, distribution, metabolism, and excretion. Researchers are examining the possibility of drug-herb interactions using laboratory and in vivo experiments as well as clinical trials, including human volunteers, in order to identify potential risks and develop guidelines for the safe and effective co-administration of herbal and conventional antiviral medications.

In summary, studies on the effectiveness of herbal antivirals offer a promising way to find new ways to treat viral infections. Researchers can clarify the mechanisms of action of herbal remedies, find new leads for antiviral medication discovery and development, and assess the safety and efficacy of medicinal plants in preclinical and clinical studies by rigorously scientifically examining them. Utilizing herbal remedies with antiviral properties reflects a synthesis of contemporary science and traditional knowledge, providing comfort and hope in the face of viral dangers to human health and adaptability.

Challenges and Limitations of Herbal Medicine Research

Research on herbal medicine, especially in the context of antiviral efficacy, must overcome some obstacles and constraints to fully utilize medicinal plants' potential in fighting viral infections. The complicated and varied chemical makeup of herbal treatments is one of the main obstacles, as it can make it challenging to repeat and standardize testing results. Hundreds or even thousands of bioactive chemicals can be found in medicinal plants, and many of these compounds can interact antagonistically or cooperatively to create therapeutic effects. Additionally, the chemical profile and biological activity of herbal treatments can be influenced by various factors, including plant species, geographical origin, growing circumstances, harvesting procedures, and processing techniques. As a result, testing results may vary. The need for uniformity and reproducibility in research investigations necessitates the standardization of herbal extracts and formulations; nevertheless, this is still a significant barrier because medicinal plants are diverse, and there are no established standards for quality control and analysis.

Lack of strong preclinical and clinical evidence to support the safety and efficacy of herbal medicines is another obstacle facing research in herbal medicine. Though they are sometimes anecdotal and lack scientific rigor, traditional knowledge and practical observations offer essential insights into the healing potential of medicinal plants. Many herbal medicines need more systematic examination in clinical studies or preclinical models, making it difficult to determine their safety, efficacy, and ideal dosage schedules. Furthermore, methodological flaws, including insufficient blinding and randomization, small sample sizes, and poor controls, might increase bias and complicate the interpretation of study results. To produce high-quality evidence that supports the use of herbal medicines in antiviral therapy and guides clinical practice, rigorous, well-designed research studies are required.

Funding and resource issues are another problem for herbal medicine research, especially compared to pharmaceutical drug development. Investment in herbal medicine research may be discouraged by the high expense and protracted development timelines of drug discovery and development, particularly for illnesses like viral infections that would not be profitable markets for pharmaceutical corporations. In addition, the regulatory landscape for herbal medications differs significantly throughout nations, with specific areas needing supervision mechanisms and explicit regulations about efficacy, safety, and quality control. Patients may have less access to herbal therapies and difficulty integrating them into traditional healthcare systems if they are not reimbursed or approved by regulations.

Research on herbal medicine is also hampered by ethical issues, mainly about biopiracy, cultural appropriation, and intellectual property rights. Indigenous knowledge and cultural practices passed down through the centuries without official recognition or remuneration for indigenous populations are at the foundation of many traditional healing systems. Without sufficient benefit-sharing agreements with indigenous peoples, researchers risk abusing traditional knowledge and biodiversity for financial gain as they work to uncover and commercialize bioactive molecules from medicinal plants. To guarantee ethical conduct in herbal medicine research and to advance equal access to the health benefits of medicinal plants, it is imperative to respect the rights, values, and sovereignty of indigenous groups.

In addition, more cooperation and multidisciplinary research are required in herbal medicine to solve methodological issues and tackle complex scientific problems. Research on herbal medicine can benefit from integrating knowledge from other domains, including pharmacognosy, phytochemistry, pharmacology, virology, immunology, and clinical medicine. Collaborative relationships among academic institutions, research organizations, industrial stakeholders, and indigenous people in herbal medicine research can promote knowledge sharing, technology transfer, and capacity building. Researchers can overcome the difficulties and constraints associated with studying herbal medicine and realize the full potential of medicinal plants in antiviral therapy by encouraging cooperation and creativity.

In summary, although herbal medicine has the potential to yield new antiviral treatments, several obstacles and restrictions need to be overcome before this field of study can reach its full potential. The advancement of herbal medicine research and its integration into mainstream healthcare practice necessitates the standardization of herbal extracts, robust preclinical and clinical studies, sufficient financing and resources, ethical considerations, and interdisciplinary collaboration. By surmounting these obstacles, scholars might leverage the potency of therapeutic plants to counteract viral infections and enhance worldwide health consequences. Utilizing herbal remedies with antiviral properties reflects a synthesis of contemporary science and traditional knowledge, providing comfort and hope in the face of viral dangers to human health and adaptability.

CHAPTER V

Common Herbal Antivirals

Overview of Key Herbal Antivirals

A review of critical herbal antivirals demonstrates a wide range of therapeutic plants with strong antiviral effects, providing encouraging choices for treating viral infections. Drawing from years of empirical knowledge and observation, traditional healers and herbalists have relied on the therapeutic potential of plants to prevent, relieve, and treat viral infections throughout history. Modern research has proven Numerous medicinal plants to be effective antiviral medicines, giving insight into their modes of action and therapeutic potential. In the face of viral threats to human health and resilience, the plant world offers a wealth of bioactive compounds with antiviral activity, ranging from herbs and spices to roots and berries. These compounds offer hope and healing.

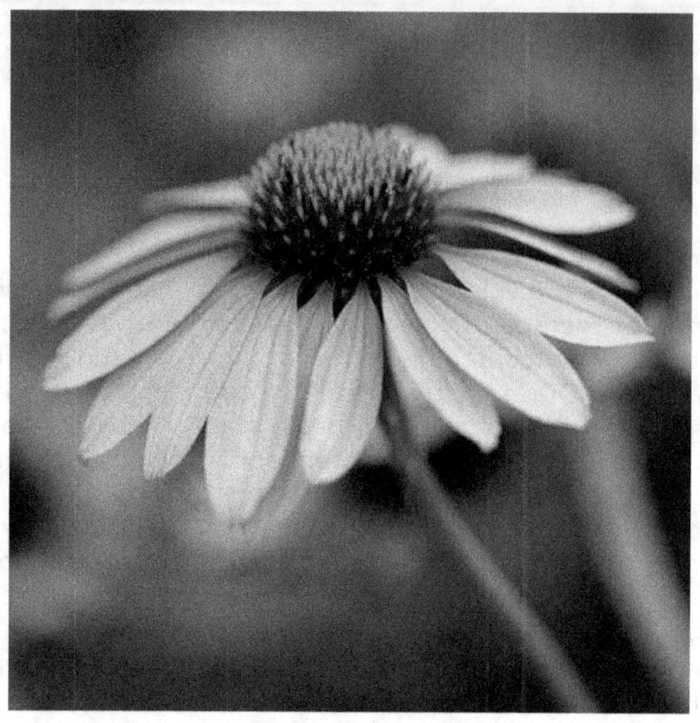

One of the most well-known herbal antivirals is echinacea
(Echinacea purpurea and Echinacea angustifolia), valued
for its immune-stimulating and antiviral qualities.
Echinacea has been demonstrated to activate the immune
system, increase white blood cell activity, and limit virus
replication—reasons why Native American tribes have
long utilized it to cure infections. Research has indicated
that echinacea extracts have the potential to mitigate the
intensity and length of colds, influenza, and other
pulmonary infections, thereby making it a well-liked
treatment for seasonal ailments.

Another potent herbal antiviral that is well-known for its
immune-modulating and anti-inflammatory properties is
elderberry (Sambucus nigra). Flavonoids found in
elderberries, such as quercetin and anthocyanins, have
been demonstrated to reduce inflammation brought on by
viral infections and prevent the multiplication of viruses.

Elderberry extracts have been shown in clinical trials to reduce the length and intensity of flu symptoms, especially when taken as soon as symptoms appear. Lozenges, tea, and elderberry syrup are frequently used to strengthen immunity and reduce symptoms of cold, flu, and other viral respiratory illnesses.

Garlic (Allium sativum) possesses antibacterial solid and immune-stimulating qualities, which have led to its use as a natural medicine for infections for millennia. Sulfur-containing substances found in garlic, such as allicin, have been demonstrated to prevent viral replication and increase the development of new immune cells. Studies indicate that garlic might help combat various viruses, such as respiratory syncytial virus (RSV), herpes simplex virus, and influenza. To prevent and treat viral infections, raw garlic or supplements containing garlic are frequently utilized by themselves or in conjunction with other antiviral herbs.

Because of its immune-modulating and antiviral properties, licorice root (Glycyrrhiza glabra) has long been used in traditional medical systems like Ayurveda and traditional Chinese medicine (TCM). Glycyrrhizin, a substance found in licorice, has been demonstrated to suppress viral replication and lessen inflammation in viral infections. According to research, licorice root extracts can prevent the spread of HIV, herpes simplex virus, and influenza, making them a viable herbal treatment for viral infections. However, because licorice can have adverse effects and interact with some drugs, it should be used cautiously.

The adaptable herb ginger (Zingiber officinale) has several therapeutic uses, including the ability to fight viruses. Bioactive substances found in ginger, such as school and gingerol, have been demonstrated to boost immune system performance and prevent the spread of viruses. Ginger might be useful in combating respiratory viruses, including coronaviruses, influenza, and respiratory syncytial virus (RSV). To strengthen immunity and reduce the symptoms of viral infections, especially those affecting the respiratory system, ginger tea, supplements, and meals flavored with ginger are frequently utilized.

Astragalus (Astragalus membranaceus), a common plant in TCM, is prized for its antiviral and immune-stimulating properties. Astragalus contains polysaccharides, saponins, and flavonoids that have been shown to enhance immune response, prevent viral replication, and reduce inflammation. Studies have shown that Astragalus extracts enhance immune responses against viral infections, especially those affecting the respiratory system. During the cold and flu season, astragalus supplements and herbal formulations are frequently used as a preventative measure to strengthen immunity and lower the risk of viral infections.

Another herbal antiviral with a long history of usage in Mediterranean and traditional herbal medicine is olive leaf (Olea europaea). Oleuropein, a substance found in olive leaves, has been demonstrated to have potent antiviral, antioxidant, and immune-modulating effects. Studies indicate that various viruses, such as the human immunodeficiency virus (HIV), herpes simplex virus, and influenza, can be inhibited from replicating by extracts from olive leaves. Supplements and tinctures made from olive leaf are commonly used to support the immune system's defense against viral infections, particularly those that impact the respiratory and gastrointestinal systems.

To sum up, a review of the essential herbal antivirals demonstrates the abundance of therapeutic plants with strong antiviral qualities, providing encouraging choices for treating viral infections. Many bioactive chemicals with potential therapeutic applications may be found in the plant world, ranging from immune-boosting herbs like echinacea and astragalus to antiviral spices like garlic and ginger. We can improve health and resilience against viral threats by utilizing the medicinal properties of plants to create herbal antiviral remedies. Using herbal remedies with antiviral properties is a way to combine traditional knowledge with contemporary research, which gives patients hope and healing when combating viral illnesses.

Properties and Mechanisms of Action

An exciting and diverse area of medicinal plant research is the properties and mechanisms of action that underlie the antiviral properties of herbal remedies. These characteristics cover a wide range of bioactive substances, each with a distinct mode of action against viral infections, that can be discovered in berries, roots, herbs, and other botanical sources. Comprehending herbal antivirals' characteristics and modes of action is crucial in clarifying their medicinal possibilities and providing guidance for creating efficacious antiviral treatments.

One of their main characteristics is the immune-modulating capabilities of herbal antivirals, which strengthen the body's natural defenses against viral infections. Bioactive components included in numerous medicinal plants, including polysaccharides, flavonoids, and saponins, promote the growth and operation of immune cells, including natural killer cells, macrophages, and T lymphocytes. These substances improve viral clearance, lessen the intensity and length of infections, and strengthen the immune response against viral pathogens. Herbal antivirals can be used therapeutically or prophylactically to treat viral diseases by modifying immune function.

The capacity of herbal antivirals to impede viral multiplication and growth within host cells is another significant characteristic. Bioactive substances found in various medicinal plants disrupt different phases of the viral replication cycle, such as virion assembly and release, protein synthesis, genome replication, and viral entrance. For example, it has been shown that polyphenols such as quercetin and epigallocatechin gallate (EGCG) prevent viruses from attaching to themselves and entering host cells, therefore stopping their growth and spread. Terpenoids like thymol and carvacrol disrupt viral membranes and stop virion particles from assembling and releasing. Terpenoids that interfere with viral membranes, such as thymol and carvacrol, prevent the assembly and release of virion particles. Herbal antivirals can lessen the severity of viral infections by interfering with viral replication and reducing the viral load by specifically targeting vital viral proteins and enzymes.

Furthermore, potent antioxidant and anti-inflammatory qualities found in herbal antivirals are essential in the fight against viral infections. Two critical processes underlie viral pathogenesis are oxidative stress and inflammation, which contribute to tissue damage, immunological dysfunction, and disease advancement.

Antioxidants like vitamin C, E, and polyphenols found in many medicinal plants scavenge free radicals and lower oxidative stress, shielding cells and tissues from harm from viral infections. Herbal antivirals can also control cytokine production and inflammatory pathways, which can limit overreactions by the immune system and lessen inflammation brought on by viral infections. Herbal antivirals help reduce inflammation and oxidative stress, improve tissue healing, and hasten the healing process from viral infections.

Herbal antivirals are also an excellent alternative for treating viral infections since they frequently show broad-spectrum effectiveness against various virus types. Herbal medicines contain a complex blend of bioactive substances that can exert pleiotropic effects against various viral infections, in contrast to conventional antiviral drugs that target specific viral proteins or enzymes. For instance, glycyrrhizin, a substance found in licorice root (Glycyrrhiza glabra), has been demonstrated to prevent the spread of HIV, herpes simplex virus, and influenza. Comparably, flavonoids found in elderberries (Sambucus nigra), such as quercetin and anthocyanins, have been shown to have antiviral properties against coronaviruses, influenza, and respiratory syncytial virus (RSV). Herbal antivirals can offer broad-spectrum protection against viral infections, lowering the risk of viral resistance and improving treatment efficacy by focusing on several phases of the viral replication cycle and modifying host immune responses.

Additionally, herbal antivirals and conventional antiviral medications frequently interact synergistically to increase the effectiveness of the former and lower the likelihood of drug resistance. Many medicinal plants' diverse bioactive chemicals can work in concert to enhance their antiviral effects. Herbal combos such as licorice root, echinacea, and elderberry have been demonstrated to improve immune function and prevent viral reproduction, offering more therapeutic advantages than any herb used alone. Researchers can create more potent combination medicines for treating viral infections by leveraging the synergistic interactions between conventional medications and herbal antivirals.

In summary, the characteristics and modes of action that underlie the antiviral effects of herbs constitute an extensive and intricate field of study with significant consequences for human health and well-being. Herbal antivirals provide diverse benefits when it comes to treating viral infections, including immune-modulating effects, prevention of viral replication and proliferation, antioxidant and anti-inflammatory qualities, broad-spectrum activity, and synergistic interactions with conventional medications. By elucidating the properties and mechanisms of action of herbal antivirals, researchers can fully leverage the therapeutic potential of medicinal plants and develop effective antiviral medications for the prophylaxis and management of viral infections. Utilizing herbal remedies with antiviral properties reflects a synthesis of contemporary science and traditional knowledge, providing comfort and hope in the face of viral dangers to human health and adaptability.

Usage and Dosage Guidelines

The effectiveness, safety, and therapeutic effects of herbal antiviral therapies depend on adherence to prescribed usage and dosage instructions. While using medicinal plants to treat viral infections can be a natural and comprehensive method, using them sensibly and by accepted practices to optimize benefits and reduce dangers is essential. Herbal treatments are available in various formats, each with specific dose guidelines and pharmacokinetic profiles, such as teas, tinctures, capsules, extracts, and topical applications. To fully utilize herbal medicine's antiviral properties, patients and healthcare professionals must comprehend the fundamentals of dosage and administration.

Individualization, which acknowledges that every person may react to herbal remedies differently depending on characteristics, including age, weight, health state, and underlying medical issues, is one of the fundamental concepts of herbal medicine dosage. Herbalists and medical professionals consider a patient's constitution, vitality, and susceptibility to infections when choosing the correct dosage and course of treatment. Variables like the type of virus, the severity and length of symptoms, and concurrent medical problems also influence dosage considerations. Herbalists can reduce side effects and maximize therapeutic results by customizing herbal treatments to each patient's unique needs and circumstances.

The idea of a minimally effective dose, which describes the smallest quantity of a medicinal plant or bioactive ingredient required to generate a therapeutic effect, is another crucial factor to consider when determining the dosage of herbal medicines. Herbalists use the lowest effective dose feasible to minimize adverse effects while maintaining medicinal efficacy. Solid herbs and bioactive substances with limited therapeutic windows or the potential to be hazardous should pay particular attention to this principle. To attain the best possible therapeutic results, practitioners can monitor each patient's response and modify the dosage by starting with low dosages and titrating up gradually as needed.

Furthermore, the form and preparation of herbal remedies and bioavailability and absorption of bioactive substances are considered when developing dose guidelines for herbal medicines. While tinctures and extracts provide a more concentrated and standardized form of herbal medicine, teas, and infusions may need longer brewing durations or higher plant concentrations to extract enough bioactive ingredients. Different dosage recommendations may apply depending on the preparation technique, strength, and planned administration route. Depending on the application area and the intensity of symptoms, different dosage considerations may be necessary for topical treatments, including creams, ointments, and poultices.

Herbal medication dose guidelines also consider the length and frequency of treatment, acknowledging that long-term, regular therapy is frequently necessary for viral infections to yield the best results. Higher dosages and more frequent application of herbal medicines may be necessary for acute infections to inhibit viral reproduction, relieve symptoms, and aid in recovery. Longer-term treatment plans may be necessary for chronic infections or repeated outbreaks to preserve immune function, stop viral reactivation, and lower the risk of consequences. To avoid resistance or desensitization to herbal medicines and to give the body a chance to recuperate, herbalists frequently advise taking periodic vacations from therapy.

Furthermore, safety is the top priority when developing dosage guidelines for herbal medicines, especially for vulnerable groups, including children, expectant mothers, people with weakened immune systems, and people with long-term medical issues. Some herbs risk adverse effects, medicine interactions, or allergic reactions when taken in large amounts or over extended periods. Before recommending herbal treatments to patients, healthcare providers and herbalists carefully evaluate the safety profile of these medicines, taking into account any contraindications and precautions. They also offer advice on parameter monitoring and toxicity indicators to guarantee the secure and efficient use of herbal antiviral treatments.

In conclusion, usage and dosage guidelines are critical to maximize herbal antiviral treatments' effectiveness, safety, and therapeutic effects. Practitioners can maximize herbal antiviral powers while minimizing risks by customizing treatment plans, utilizing the lowest effective dose, taking into account the form and preparation of herbal remedies, deciding on the length and frequency of treatment, and prioritizing safety concerns. Integrating herbal remedies into mainstream healthcare requires several critical measures, including educating patients and healthcare providers about responsible use of herbal medicines and offering evidence-based dosage recommendations. Utilizing herbal remedies with antiviral properties reflects a synthesis of contemporary science and traditional knowledge, providing comfort and hope in the face of viral dangers to human health and adaptability.

CHAPTER VI

Integrating Herbal and Conventional Medicine

Understanding the Synergy Between Herbal and Conventional Treatments

Comprehending the mutual benefits between herbal and conventional treatments is essential to contemporary healthcare, especially when fighting viral infections. Herbal treatments provide an alternative to conventional antiviral medications, which can improve therapeutic results, limit side effects, and lower the likelihood of drug resistance. Conventional antiviral medications are still essential for treating viral diseases. Healthcare professionals can create comprehensive and individualized treatment plans that address the complicated nature of viral infections and promote maximum health and wellness by integrating the benefits of both herbal and conventional treatments.

The complementing mechanisms of action of herbal and conventional treatments against viral viruses are one of the main advantages of integrating them. Typically, specific viral proteins or enzymes involved in viral assembly, replication, or entrance into host cells are the targets of conventional antiviral medications. Conversely, various bioactive chemicals found in herbal treatments can modify host immune responses and exert pleiotropic effects against different stages of the viral replication cycle. Healthcare professionals can lower the likelihood of virus resistance and increase overall antiviral efficacy by combining medications with distinct mechanisms of action. Herbal medicines, such as licorice root (Glycyrrhiza glabra) and elderberry (Sambucus nigra), have demonstrated the ability to impede virus replication and improve immune function. As such, they can be a supplementary treatment to traditional antiviral medications.

Additionally, synergistic interactions between herbal and conventional medicines enhance their antiviral efficacy. Many medicinal plants include bioactive chemicals that, by modifying medication metabolism, absorption, distribution, and excretion, can improve the pharmacokinetics, bioavailability, and efficacy of conventional pharmaceuticals. For instance, herbs like turmeric (Curcuma longa) and ginger (Zingiber officinale) have been demonstrated to improve drug absorption and slow down metabolism, boosting bioavailability and extending therapeutic benefits. Healthcare professionals can maximize drug delivery, improve therapeutic outcomes, and reduce adverse effects by mixing herbal therapies with conventional medications.

Additionally, a comprehensive and individualized approach to managing viral infections is made possible by combining herbal and conventional treatments, considering each patient's health status, preferences, and treatment objectives. Herbal treatments provide patients with a more integrated and patient-centered approach to healthcare with an all-natural, comprehensive alternative to prescription medications. Healthcare professionals can customize treatment plans to match each patient's unique needs and circumstances by considering the patient's constitution, vitality, and susceptibility to infections. This helps to maximize therapeutic outcomes and support long-term health and wellness.

Furthermore, by combining herbal and conventional treatments, medical professionals can target different components of the disease process at the same time and address the multifaceted character of viral infections. Treatment for viral infections must be extensive and multifaceted since the virus, host immune system and environmental variables frequently interact in complex ways. In addition to the specific action of conventional antiviral medications, herbal medicines provide a wide range of bioactive components that can alter immune function, reduce inflammation, and accelerate tissue healing. Healthcare practitioners can expedite healing, lower the risk of complications, and enhance overall health outcomes by addressing viral infections' root causes and contributing factors.

Additionally, by giving people a wide range of therapeutic options to manage their health and well-being, the integration of herbal and conventional treatments encourages patient empowerment and self-care. Due to the fact that many herbal medications may be made at home or purchased over the counter, patients are better equipped to actively control their health. Teaching patients about the benefits and drawbacks of both conventional and herbal medicines might enable people to make well-informed choices about their treatments and participate more actively in their healthcare journeys.

Furthermore, integrating herbal treatments into conventional medical practice fosters greater inclusivity and equity in healthcare access and delivery by promoting cultural diversity, traditional knowledge, and sustainability.

Knowing how herbal and conventional therapies work in concert provides a potent strategy for treating viral infections and fostering the best possible health and wellness. Healthcare professionals may create complete and individualized treatment plans that address the complexity of viral infections, improve therapeutic outcomes, and give patients the confidence to actively control their health by integrating the strengths of both modalities. In the face of viral threats to human health and resilience, harnessing the synergy between herbal and conventional medicines symbolizes a synthesis of traditional wisdom and modern science, providing hope and healing.

Collaboration Between Herbalists and Modern Healthcare Practitioners

Integrating traditional therapeutic techniques into mainstream healthcare and the full potential of herbal antiviral properties can be achieved through collaboration between herbalists and contemporary healthcare practitioners. Herbalists provide invaluable insights into the therapeutic qualities, mechanisms of action, and safety issues of herbal treatments because of their extensive understanding of medicinal plants and traditional healing methods. Their knowledge is founded on centuries of clinical experience and practical observation, which offers a solid basis for comprehending the therapeutic benefits of medicinal plants. On the other hand, contemporary medical professionals offer clinical knowledge, scientific rigor, and access to cutting-edge diagnostic equipment and instruments that can improve our comprehension of and confidence in herbal medicine for treating viral infections. Herbalists and contemporary healthcare professionals can bridge the gap between conventional wisdom and scientific innovation by working together and exchanging knowledge. This will enable patients to receive more individualized and comprehensive care for viral infections and better overall health and wellness.

Collaboration between herbalists and contemporary healthcare practitioners offers several advantages, including sharing knowledge and skills and leveraging the advantages of both traditional and evidence-based medicine. Herbalists are deeply knowledgeable in traditional therapeutic methods, botanical preparations, and medicinal plants passed down through the years.

Drawing from decades of empirical observation and clinical experience, they provide invaluable insights into herbal treatments' medicinal characteristics, mechanisms of action, and safety issues. Conversely, contemporary medical professionals offer clinical knowledge, scientific rigor, and access to cutting-edge diagnostic equipment and technology that can improve our comprehension of and confidence in using herbal medicine in the setting of viral infections.

Furthermore, herbalists and contemporary medical professionals can work together to provide a more integrative and holistic approach to patient care that considers the patient's mental, emotional, physical, and spiritual well-being. Herbalists frequently take a holistic approach to health and illness, considering the connection between the mind, body, and spirit and correcting underlying imbalances or disease's underlying causes. To promote health and avoid sickness, they strongly emphasize the role that lifestyle factors play, including nutrition, exercise, stress reduction, and environmental factors. Modern healthcare professionals can provide patients with a more thorough and individualized approach to controlling viral infections and boosting general health and wellness by incorporating herbal treatments into standard healthcare practice.

Additionally, by acknowledging other communities' and cultures' many viewpoints, beliefs, and healing customs, cooperation between herbalists and contemporary healthcare professionals promotes better inclusivity and cultural competence in healthcare delivery. Herbal medicine originates in indigenous knowledge and cultural practices, which reflect the world's varied peoples' spiritual ties, stewardship of the environment, and distinctive biodiversity. Modern healthcare professionals may improve healthcare access and equity by respecting and honoring traditional healing traditions and developing partnerships, rapport, and trust with marginalized groups and indigenous communities.

Furthermore, cooperation between contemporary healthcare professionals and herbalists promotes research and innovation in herbal medicine, expanding the evidence supporting its safety, effectiveness, and uses in clinical settings. The therapeutic effects of medicinal plants can be better understood through empirical observations and traditional knowledge. Still, rigorous scientific study is required to confirm their effectiveness, clarify their mechanisms of action, and guide evidence-based therapy. Collaborative research projects involving scientists, herbalists, and healthcare organizations can conduct clinical trials, systematic reviews, and meta-analyses of herbal remedies for viral infections. These projects can take advantage of the advantages of both traditional knowledge and contemporary science.

Herbalists and contemporary healthcare professionals working together also support the sustainability and conservation of medicinal plants, emphasizing the value of ethical sourcing, biodiversity, and environmental stewardship in herbal medicine. Numerous medicinal plants are at risk to biodiversity and world health due to habitat loss, overharvesting, climate change, and unsustainable harvesting methods. Herbalists and contemporary healthcare providers can preserve traditional knowledge, protect endangered species, and promote local economies by encouraging the sustainable cultivation, harvesting, and trading medicinal plants.

Working together, herbalists and contemporary medical professionals might unlock the potential of herbal antiviral properties and incorporate conventional healing methods into medical practice. Herbalists and contemporary healthcare practitioners can collaborate to improve healthcare access, equity, and outcomes by sharing knowledge and expertise, taking a holistic and integrative approach to patient care, encouraging inclusivity and cultural competence, advancing research and innovation, and promoting sustainability and conservation. In the face of infectious threats to human health and well-being, harnessing the synergy between traditional wisdom and contemporary science offers a potent route to healing and resistance.

Case Studies: Successful Integrative Approaches

Case studies that demonstrate effective integrative methods for utilizing the antiviral properties of herbs provide insightful information about the possible advantages of fusing conventional medical therapies with traditional therapeutic methods. These case studies show how working with modern healthcare practitioners and herbalists can improve patient happiness and therapeutic outcomes and advance holistic health and wellness. Healthcare professionals can provide patients with a comprehensive and efficient plan for managing viral infections and promoting general well-being by incorporating herbal treatments into standard medical practice and using a tailored, patient-centered approach to treatment.

In one case study, a patient with recurrent herpes simplex virus (HSV) infections is treated with herbal therapies and traditional antiviral medications. The 35-year-old patient had been taking antiviral drugs as directed by her primary care physician, but she continued to have recurrent outbreaks of oral herpes. She saw an herbalist searching for other therapeutic options, and the herbalist suggested a concoction of echinacea, licorice root, and lemon balm— herbal treatments well-known for their antiviral and immune-boosting qualities. The herbalist and the patient's medical team created a customized treatment plan that included herbal therapies and traditional antiviral medications. The patient experienced an improvement in her general well-being and quality of life after only a few weeks of beginning the herbal therapy regimen. She also reported a considerable decrease in the frequency and severity of her herpes episodes.

An additional case study demonstrates the effective incorporation of herbal medicine in treating a pediatric patient's influenza. A 6-year-old child with symptoms of fever, cough, and sore throat suggestive of influenza infection was brought into the emergency room. The child's parents, who supported holistic medicine, stated that they would like to look into alternative therapies in addition to traditional medical ones. The medical staff worked with an herbalist who suggested ginger tea, astragalus, garlic, and elderberry syrup. As the medical staff kept an eye on the child's symptoms and clinical development, the herbalist offered advice on dose, administration, and safety issues. In contrast to prior influenza occurrences, the child's symptoms were quickly resolved, and his sickness lasted less time, thanks to the integrative approach, which demonstrated the potential advantages of integrating herbal medicines with traditional medical care.

Moreover, the therapy of a chronic hepatitis C virus (HCV) infection case study highlights the function of herbal medicine in promoting the immune system and liver health. In addition to antiviral medication and routine liver function testing, a 45-year-old man with a persistent HCV infection looked for complementary alternative therapies. The patient saw an herbalist, who suggested dietary and lifestyle changes to boost detoxification pathways and lessen liver inflammation, along with a combination of hepatoprotective herbs like milk thistle, dandelion root, and schizandra berry. The herbalist collaborated with the patient's medical team to ensure the herbal medicines were secure and in line with the patient's traditional treatment plan. The integration of herbal therapy with conventional medical care can be beneficial in managing persistent viral infections. The patient's quality of life was improved, liver function tests were better, and the viral load was decreased over time due to the integrative approach.

Finally, case studies demonstrating effective integrative methods for utilizing the antiviral properties of herbs illustrate the potential advantages of fusing conventional medical interventions with traditional therapeutic methods. Healthcare professionals can provide patients with a comprehensive and efficient plan for managing viral infections and promoting general well-being by incorporating herbal treatments into standard medical practice and using a tailored, patient-centered approach to treatment. Herbalists and contemporary healthcare professionals working together can lead to better therapeutic results, happier patients, and more holistic health and wellness. In the face of infectious threats to human health and well-being, harnessing the synergy between traditional wisdom and contemporary science offers a potent route to healing and resistance.

CHAPTER VII

Herbal Antivirals in Practice

Building Your Herbal Antiviral Toolkit

Choosing and combining various medicinal plants and botanical preparations with strong antiviral effects is part of creating your herbal antiviral toolkit. You may strengthen your immune system, increase your resistance to viral infections, and advance general health and well-being by compiling an extensive toolset of herbal medicines. However, as incorrect use or dosage of medicinal plants can have adverse effects, it is imperative to approach herbal medicine with caution, respect, and education. You can assemble a secure and efficient herbal antiviral toolkit that suits your unique requirements and tastes with thorough research, expert herbalist advice, and consultation with medical specialists.

Immune-boosting herbs are vital to your herbal antiviral repertoire since they support your body's natural defenses against viral infections. These herbs boost immunity, increase immune cell generation and activity, and increase resistance to pathogenic pathogens. Herbs that support the immune system include elderberry (Sambucus nigra), astragalus (Astragalus membranaceous), and echinacea (Echinacea purpurea).

Astragalus is valued for its capacity to improve immune function and foster infection resistance, whereas echinacea is well known for its immune-stimulating qualities. It has been demonstrated that elderberries, which are high in flavonoids and antioxidants, lessen the intensity and length of viral infections like the flu and colds.

Furthermore, antiviral herbs are vital additions to your repertoire since they target viral pathogens and prevent their multiplication. These herbs have bioactive ingredients that disrupt the viral replication cycle at different points: virion assembly and release, protein synthesis, genome replication, and viral entry. Herbs that have antiviral properties include garlic (Allium sativum), lemon balm (Melissa officinalis), and licorice root (Glycyrrhiza glabra). It has been shown that licorice root, which contains a compound called glycyrrhizin, inhibits the spread of HIV, herpes simplex virus, and influenza. Garlic has broad-spectrum effectiveness against viral infections, while lemon balm has antiviral solid qualities against herpes viruses.

Moreover, anti-inflammatory herbs are a great addition to your herbal repertoire since they lessen inflammation and ease the symptoms of viral infections. A typical characteristic of viral infections is inflammation, which can aid in developing the disease, tissue damage, and immunological dysfunction. Herbs that reduce inflammation can limit overactive immune responses, regulate inflammatory pathways, and aid tissue healing and repair. Turmeric (Curcuma longa), ginger (Zingiber officinale), and Boswellia (Boswellia serrata) are a few examples of anti-inflammatory herbs. Curcumin, a potent anti-inflammatory found in turmeric, has been demonstrated to lessen inflammation and ease the symptoms of respiratory infections. Due to their comparable anti-inflammatory qualities, ginger and Boswellia are helpful treatments for lowering fever, discomfort, and inflammation brought on by viral infections.

Additionally, adaptogenic herbs are a great addition to your herbal antiviral repertoire since they promote resilience to stress and general wellness. Adaptogens increase energy levels, support equilibrium and homeostasis, and assist the body in adjusting to psychological, physiological, and environmental stimuli. Herbs like rhodiola (Rhodiola rosea), holy basil (Ocimum sanctum), and ashwagandha (Withania somnifera) are examples of adaptogenic herbs. Also referred to as "Indian ginseng," ashwagandha supports immune system function, enhances resilience against infections, and modulates the stress response. While holy basil supports relaxation, mental well-being, and immune resilience, Rhodiola increases energy, mental clarity, and physical endurance.

Additionally, you can increase the overall efficacy of your herbal antiviral toolkit by using supporting herbs that support and improve particular organ systems or bodily functions. These herbs offer specific assistance for digestive, circulatory, respiratory, and other physiological processes impacted by viral infections. Herbs that are considered supportive include milk thistle (Silybum marianum) for liver health, mullein (Verbascum thapsus) for respiratory health, ginger, and peppermint (Mentha piperita) for digestive health, and hawthorn (Crataegus spp.) for cardiovascular health. You can treat underlying imbalances or weaknesses and promote holistic health and wellness by adding supportive herbs to your herbal repertoire.

To summarize, creating an herbal antiviral toolkit entails choosing and utilizing various medicinal plants and botanical preparations with antiviral solid, immune-stimulating, anti-inflammatory, adaptogenic, and supporting features. Build a complete arsenal of herbal treatments specific to your needs and tastes, and you may boost your immune system, strengthen your defenses against viral infections, and advance general health and well-being. For the secure and efficient consumption of plants for medicinal purposes, it is imperative to approach herbal medicine with caution, respect, and experience. Qualified herbalists and healthcare professionals can provide valuable help in this regard. To safeguard yourself and your loved ones against viral health risks, you may assemble a powerful and efficient herbal antiviral toolkit with thorough study, well-informed decision-making, and a dedication to holistic health.

Practical Tips for Incorporating Herbal Remedies into Daily Life

Using herbal treatments in daily life can lead to holistic health and wellness in a fulfilling and empowering way. Herbal medicine offers a wide range of botanical preparations and traditional healing techniques that can enrich and supplement your daily routine, whether your goals are to manage stress, strengthen your immune system, or promote overall vitality. Through the deliberate and intelligent incorporation of herbal medicines into your lifestyle, you can effectively utilize the medical properties of plants while fostering a stronger bond with the natural world, self-care, and overall well- being. The following helpful advice can help you incorporate herbal treatments into your day-to-day routine:

To begin with, familiarize yourself with the characteristics, applications, and safety measures of various medicinal plants and botanical medicines. Spend time investigating reliable sources, speaking with knowledgeable herbalists or medical experts, and perusing reliable books, websites, and instructional materials on herbal medicine. You can make well-informed choices about herbs to include in your daily routine and how to use them safely and efficiently by laying a solid foundation of knowledge and understanding.

Secondly, try various herbal concoctions and cures to see which suits you best. Herbal medicine provides various possibilities, each with specific benefits and applications.

These options include teas, tinctures, capsules, extracts, essential oils, and topical preparations. Try a few basic remedies, such as herbal teas for relaxation, tinctures for immune support, or fragrant herbs for stress relief, to see which ones work best for your health objectives and personal preferences. Based on your unique demands and experiences, pay attention to how your body reacts to each cure and modify your choices accordingly.

Thirdly, include herbal medicines sustainably and regularly in your everyday practice. To fully reap the therapeutic advantages of herbs and integrate herbal medicine into your daily routine, look for methods to incorporate them into your meals, drinks, self-care routines, and housework routines. Herbal tinctures or extracts can strengthen the immune system, dried or fresh herbs can be added to food, herbal infusions or essential oils can be used to make homemade skincare products, and herbal teas can be brewed for relaxation and hydration. By incorporating herbal remedies into your everyday routines and habits, you can strengthen your sense of self-care and connection to nature, as well as improve your general health and wellness.

Fourthly, quality and sustainability are prioritized when procuring botanical preparations and herbal treatments. To guarantee their purity, potency, and ecological integrity, choose organic herbs and botanicals that are responsibly farmed and sustainably obtained whenever feasible. Seek trustworthy growers, manufacturers, and suppliers who follow strict guidelines for environmental responsibility, quality assurance, and openness in their farming, harvesting, processing, and distribution methods. You may aid in conserving biodiversity and medicinal plants while advancing the health and well-being of people and ecosystems worldwide by supporting the herbal industry's ethical and sustainable business practices.

Fifth, when utilizing herbal medicines, pay attention to your body and believe in your instincts. Honor your body's wisdom and input by observing how different herbs make you feel physically, emotionally, and energetic. Trust your intuition and look into more possibilities that better fit your needs and preferences if a particular herb doesn't speak to you or has negative consequences. Similarly, if a particular herb is helping you, keep using it in your daily routine and discover its potential to help you on your path to better health and fitness.

Finally, as you start your herbal medicine journey, seek advice and support from knowledgeable herbalists, medical experts, and local resources. Never be afraid to ask questions, seek guidance, and share your experiences with others interested in natural healing methods and herbal medicines. Enrolling in herbalism courses, seminars, or support groups can offer beneficial chances for education, networking, and cooperation with like-minded people who share a passion for holistic health and herbal therapy. With courage, curiosity, and friendship, you can successfully negotiate the difficulties of herbal medicine by assembling a solid network of peers, mentors, and allies.

To sum up, using herbal remedies daily is an exploration, experimentation, and self-discovery path with many advantages for health, energy, and wellness. You can harness the medicinal powers of plants and cultivate a deeper connection to nature, self-care, and holistic well-being by educating yourself, trying out different remedies, incorporating herbs into your daily routine, prioritizing quality and sustainability, listening to your body, and seeking support from knowledgeable herbalists and healthcare professionals. You can embark on a life-changing herbal medicine journey that nourishes your body, mind, and spirit while encouraging resilience, balance, and vigor in all facets of your life if you approach it with thoughtful intention and an open mind.

Recipes and Formulations for Herbal Antiviral Preparations

Herbal antiviral preparation recipes and formulas provide helpful and approachable methods to use medicinal plants' healing properties to fight viral infections. A wide range of herbal preparations can be included in daily living to improve immune function, increase resilience, and enhance general well-being. These include immune-boosting beverages, calming herbal tinctures, and powerful topical medicines. People can participate actively in their health and healing by experimenting with different recipes and formulations to tailor their herbal treatments to their unique needs, preferences, and health objectives.

Herbal tea blends are a well-liked and adaptable herbal remedy for boosting immune system performance and preventing viral infections. Typically, these mixes include flavor-enhancing and medicinally beneficial herbs like ginger, cinnamon, and lemon balm, together with immune-boosting herbs like echinacea, elderberry, and astragalus. You must steep a blend of fresh or dried herbs in hot water for five to ten minutes, filter, and drink your immune-boosting herbal tea. You can modify the amounts of the herbs in your tea blend to fit your tastes and desired potency, considering your health requirements and taste preferences.

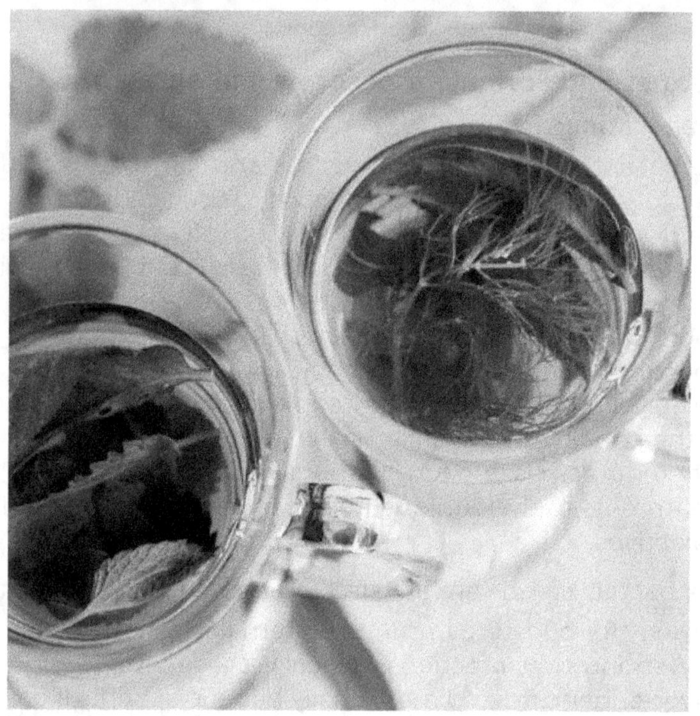

Herbal tinctures or extracts are another potent herbal preparation for antiviral support. Tinctures are potent liquid extracts created by steeping fresh or dried plants in glycerin or alcohol to release their therapeutic qualities. Herbal tinctures combine your preferred herbs with glycerin or alcohol in a glass jar, sealing it snugly and allowing it to soak for a few weeks while shaking it periodically to guarantee complete extraction. After preparing the tincture, filter the herbs out and store the liquid extract in a dark glass bottle for later use. Herbal tinctures are easy and portable for immune support when traveling because you can take them orally by adding a few drops to juice or water.

Additionally, topical treatments for viral infections and promoting skin health are provided via herbal-infused oils and salves. To produce infused oils, one must steep fresh or dried herbs in a carrier oil, such as coconut or olive oil, to extract their medicinal properties. Pack your preferred herbs into a glass jar, cover it with a carrier oil, and steep for a few weeks, shaking the jar frequently to ensure complete infusion to create a herbal-infused oil. When the oil is ready to use topically, filter the herbs out and keep the infused oil in a dark glass bottle. For calming relief from viral symptoms like rashes, itching, or inflammation, herbal-infused oils can be administered topically or used as a base for salves, balms, or massage oils.

Herbal steam inhalations also relieve congestion brought on by viral infections and support the respiratory system. To open up the airways, relax the respiratory tissues, and encourage better breathing, steam inhalations use fresh or dried herbs—like peppermint, thyme, and eucalyptus— added to hot water. To make a herbal steam inhalation, place a few herbs in a basin of hot water, cover your head with a towel, and breathe deeply for five to ten minutes. A few drops of essential oils, notably lavender, tea tree, or eucalyptus, added to the water can further improve the therapeutic benefits of steam inhalations by providing additional respiratory support and antibacterial activity.

Moreover, herbal mouthwashes and gargles provide natural treatments for lowering inflammation, relieving sore throats, and warding off mouth and throat viral infections. Antiviral herbs with antimicrobial, anti-inflammatory, and calming qualities, like licorice root, sage, and thyme, can make mouthwashes and gargles.

To use as a mouthwash or gargle, simply steep a few herbs in hot water for ten to fifteen minutes, strain, and allow the liquid to cool to room temperature. For extra flavor and health advantages, mix a few drops of honey or a grain of salt into the mouthwash. To ease sore throats and mouth discomfort, gargle or swish the herbal solution in your mouth for thirty to sixty seconds, then spit it out. Repeat as necessary.

To sum up, herbal antiviral preparation recipes and formulations provide practical and approachable means of utilizing medicinal plants' curative properties to fight viral infections and enhance general health and well-being. Herbal medicines that strengthen immune function, relieve symptoms, and improve resilience range widely and can be easily incorporated into daily life. These include immune-boosting teas and tinctures, soothing topical therapies, and respiratory steam inhalations. Through experimentation with various recipes and formulations and customization to personal tastes and requirements, people can harness the transformational potential of herbal medicine to take control of their health and healing.

CHAPTER VIII

Safety and Regulation

Ensuring Safety in Herbal Medicine Use

To maximize the therapeutic benefits of medicinal plants while lowering the danger of side effects or interactions, it is essential to ensure safety when using herbal medicines. Although using herbal treatments to support health and well-being has been done for ages, using them wisely, respectfully, and with knowledge is crucial. People can experience the healing powers of nature and safely include herbal medicine into their wellness routine without sacrificing their health or well-being by adopting informed practices and adhering to fundamental rules.

Knowing the characteristics, effects, and possible dangers of various medicinal plants is essential to guaranteeing safety when using them as herbal remedies. Not all herbs are suitable for everyone; some can worsen underlying medical issues, be combined with drugs, or have adverse side effects if taken incorrectly. It is crucial to investigate any herbal cure's qualities, applications, warnings, and possible adverse effects before using it. If necessary, get advice from qualified herbalists or medical specialists. You can reduce the possibility of problems or unfavorable reactions by educating yourself about the safety concerns and the herbs you intend to use.

Furthermore, sourcing and quality play a crucial role in guaranteeing the security and effectiveness of herbal treatments. It's crucial to select premium, ethically sourced herbs from reliable distributors, growers, and manufacturers to guarantee their potency, purity, and medicinal value. Seek organic, sustainably collected herbs subjected to independent testing and that follow strict quality control guidelines with openness in their cultivation, harvesting, processing, and distribution methods. You can reduce the possibility of contamination, adulteration, or mislabeling and ensure you're using secure and efficient herbal medicines that promote your health and well-being by prioritizing quality and sourcing.

Furthermore, appropriate administration and dose are crucial factors in guaranteeing the safety of using herbal medicines. Although, when taken as directed, herbal therapies are generally thought to be harmless, overdosing or incorrect dosage can have hazardous or adverse effects. To guarantee tolerance and efficacy, it is crucial to go by suggested dosage guidelines, start with modest dosages, progressively increase as needed, and pay attention to your body's reaction. Consult a knowledgeable herbalist or medical practitioner for advice and suggestions specific to your requirements and situation if you need clarification about using or administering a particular herb.

Furthermore, maintaining the safety of herbal medicines requires knowledge of possible interactions between herbs, prescription drugs, and other supplements. Certain herbs can modify the body's effects, metabolism, or absorption when combined with other herbs or drugs. Knowing the possibility of herb-drug interactions is crucial. If you take any prescriptions or have underlying medical issues that herbal therapies could impact, you should speak with a healthcare provider. You can prevent adverse outcomes and guarantee safe and efficient integrative care by telling your healthcare practitioner you use herbal medicines and discussing any possible interactions.

Furthermore, maintaining the safety of herbal medicines requires acknowledging the strength and efficacy of these therapies. Despite naturally occurring materials generated from plants, herbs also include bioactive chemicals with physiological solid effects. Herbal treatments should be used mindfully, sensibly, and with respect. Excessive or careless use could have unfavorable consequences or imbalances. Pay attention to your body's signals, start with modest dosages, and increase gradually as necessary. Additionally, you can start with a lower dosage and adjust how much you use according to how you feel. With knowledge and intention, you can use the therapeutic qualities of herbs to maintain balance and harmony in your body and mind.

Furthermore, preserving the safety and potency of herbal treatments over time requires the practice of correct handling and storage. Store herbs in a dark, cold spot away from heat, moisture, and sunshine to keep them fresh, potent, and medicinal. To keep herbs safe from air, moisture, and pollutants, store them in airtight jars or containers and mark them properly with the name of the herb, the date of purchase, and the expiration date. Your herbal treatments should be safe, effective, and delightful for months or years to come. This may be ensured with proper handling and storage.

In conclusion, understanding the strength and potency of medicinal plants, practicing awareness, and using herbal medicines safely are all necessary. People can safely incorporate herbal medicine into their wellness routine and feel the healing powers of nature with confidence and peace of mind by knowing the qualities, actions, and potential risks of herbs, prioritizing quality and sourcing, adhering to recommended dosage guidelines, being aware of potential interactions; respecting the potency of herbal remedies; and practicing proper storage and handling. When utilized sensibly and intelligently, herbal medicine can be a valuable tool in enhancing health, vitality, and well-being for individuals all over the world.

Regulatory Framework for Herbal Products

Herbal product regulations are essential for guaranteeing the efficacy, safety, and quality of medicinal plants and botanical preparations. As the demand for herbal medicine grows, governments worldwide have established several laws and guidelines to control the manufacturing, promotion, and sale of herbal products while preserving consumer rights and public health. These legal frameworks seek to safeguard consumers from potential risks related to the use of herbal treatments while also supporting access to traditional healing methods.

Product licensing and registration are essential to the legal system governing herbal products. Herbal products must pass stringent inspection and approval procedures in many nations before being sold and advertised to the general public. Usually, this entails sending thorough records containing proof of efficacy, safety, and quality to regulatory bodies for examination and approval. Goods that fulfill predetermined standards and requirements are granted licensing or registration, which enables them to be sold with prescribed indications, dosage guidelines, and labeling specifications. Regulatory bodies can guarantee that herbal products fulfill minimal safety and quality standards and give customers accurate information about their uses and benefits by mandating product registration and licensing.

Furthermore, an integral part of the regulatory framework for herbal goods is quality control and good manufacturing standards (GMP). To guarantee uniformity, purity, and potency throughout the production process, GMP guidelines set standards and protocols for the cultivation, harvesting, processing, packing, and labeling of medicinal plants and botanical preparations. To reduce the possibility of contamination, adulteration, or mislabeling and to preserve the integrity and safety of herbal products from the point of origin of raw materials to the point of distribution, manufacturers must abide by GMP principles. Regulatory agencies audit and inspect manufacturing facilities to ensure that GMP regulations are followed and take enforcement action against businesses that don't adhere to the rules.

Furthermore, rules governing labeling and packaging are essential for giving customers correct information about herbal products and how to utilize them. Herbal items must have labels that provide the following details: product name, ingredients, dosing guidelines, warnings, precautions, and storage requirements. The labels must be clear and easy to read. Along with the batch number, expiration date, and any applicable warnings or disclaimers, labels must also contain information about the producer or distributor. When herbal items are packaged and labeled correctly, customers are empowered to make knowledgeable decisions about their use and how to utilize them safely. Regulatory bodies enforce packaging and labeling requirements by product testing, inspections, and enforcement actions against companies that violate the regulations.

Furthermore, post-market surveillance and adverse event reporting mechanisms are crucial elements of the herbal product regulatory framework. Regulatory bodies monitor their safety and effectiveness after herbal products are licensed for marketing and usage. They do this by gathering and evaluating reports of adverse occurrences, side effects, and problems with product quality from producers, consumers, and healthcare professionals. To safeguard public health and safety, post-market surveillance assists in identifying new safety issues, spotting patterns of unfavorable reactions, and implementing the necessary regulatory measures. Regarding herbal goods, regulatory bodies have the authority to issue warnings, recalls, or product withdrawals in cases where the items pose serious dangers or do not fulfill set safety and quality criteria.

Moreover, the regulatory framework for herbal goods considers international cooperation and harmonization. Harmonizing regulatory standards and practices across nations can ease the free movement of herbal goods while maintaining consistent protection of public health and consumer rights, particularly given the global character of the trade and commerce in herbal medicines. Global standards, best practices, and recommendations are being developed for the regulation of herbal products by international organizations, including the World Healthcare Organization (WHO) and the International Organization for the Harmonization of Technical Standards for Pharmaceuticals for Human Use (ICH). International harmonization efforts aim to improve transparency, efficiency, and effectiveness of herbal product regulation globally by encouraging cooperation and mutual recognition of regulatory frameworks.

To sum up, the regulatory structure of herbal items is essential for guaranteeing the security, excellence, and potency of medicinal plants and botanical concoctions. Regulatory agencies strive to safeguard public health and consumer rights while facilitating access to traditional healing methods through product registration and licensing, quality control and GMP requirements, labeling and packaging regulations, post-market surveillance, and international harmonization efforts. Regulatory frameworks help advance the integration of herbal medicine into conventional healthcare systems, promote innovation, and increase consumer confidence by providing clear standards and procedures for producing, marketing, and distributing herbal products. Governments and stakeholders may guarantee that herbal products achieve the highest safety, quality, and efficacy standards, benefiting individuals, communities, and societies globally by continuing to collaborate and demonstrating a commitment to regulatory excellence.

Responsible Herbal Medicine Practices

Various rules and standards are included in responsible herbal medicine practices to guarantee the ethical, safe, and efficient use of medicinal plants and botanical preparations. Growing public interest in herbal therapy necessitates ethical practices that prioritize patient safety, quality control, and sustainability for individuals, practitioners, and regulatory bodies. Stakeholders may conserve the rich legacy of botanical healing for future generations, advance public health, and build confidence in herbal medicines by adopting responsible practices.

Education and training are essential components of responsible herbal medicine practices. Both individuals and practitioners of herbal medicine should pursue thorough education and training to acquire the competencies, abilities, and information required for safe and efficient practice. This can include formal education courses covering plant identification, herbal pharmacology, therapeutic applications, safety issues, and ethical principles; these can also be workshops, seminars, apprenticeships, or independent study courses.

To ensure they give their patients competent and informed care, practitioners can stay current on new research, best practices, and regulatory developments in herbal medicine by investing in ongoing education and training.

Furthermore, using herbal medicine responsibly requires dedication to critical thinking and evidence-based decision-making. Herbal medicine relies heavily on traditional knowledge and anecdotal evidence, but scientific research and clinical data must also be included to inform clinical practice and decision-making.

Practitioners must conduct a critical assessment of the caliber and dependability of research studies, appraise the degree of evidence bolstering herbal therapies, and incorporate guidelines and suggestions derived from empirical research into their treatment procedures. Herbal medicine practitioners can uphold patient-centered care and informed consent while bolstering the validity, efficacy, and credibility of botanical healing by integrating evidence-based practice.

Informed consent and collaborative decision-making are essential aspects of responsible herbal medicine practices. To enable patients to make knowledgeable decisions regarding their health and well-being, practitioners should be forthright and honest with patients regarding the possible risks, advantages, and additional options associated with herbal therapy. This entails answering any queries, worries, or preferences that patients may have and giving them precise and understandable information regarding the benefits, drawbacks, anticipated results, and possible adverse effects of herbal treatments. Practitioners can increase patient satisfaction and adherence to treatment regimens, promote autonomy, and establish trust by cultivating a respectful and cooperative relationship with their patients.

In addition, ethical production and distribution practices for herbal medicines place a high priority on quality assurance and safety throughout the whole supply chain, from harvesting and production to manufacturing and distribution. To guarantee herbal medicines' purity, potency, and safety, practitioners and manufacturers should abide by strict quality control standards, good agriculture and collection practices (GACP), and good manufacturing practices (GMP). This could entail putting quality assurance procedures into place, regularly testing and analyzing raw materials and completed goods, and following legal specifications for labeling, packaging, and marketing. Practitioners and manufacturers can reduce the possibility of contamination, adulteration, or mislabeling and offer consumers trustworthy and efficient herbal medicines by emphasizing safety and quality assurance.

Additionally, using herbal medicine responsibly means being mindful of the environment and devoted to sustainability. It is crucial to grow and harvest herbs sustainably and morally to maintain biodiversity, safeguard ecosystems, and respect local populations' rights and way of life in light of the rising demand for medicinal plants. This could entail advocating for fair trade values, sustainable farming methods, and regulations for wildcrafting in addition to supporting community-based programs that encourage the sustainable use of medicinal plants and conservation, habitat restoration, and conservation activities. Herbal medicine practitioners and stakeholders can ensure the availability and accessibility of medicinal plants for future generations while supporting the long-term health and resilience of ecosystems and communities by adopting sustainable methods.

The ethical, safe, and efficient use of therapeutic plants and botanical preparations depends on responsible herbal medicine practices. Informed consent and shared decision-making, safety and quality assurance, education and training, sustainability and environmental stewardship, evidence-informed practice, public health, and the rich legacy of botanical healing can all be preserved for future generations by practitioners and stakeholders by adhering to these principles. Herbal medicine can continue to be a valuable tool for promoting resilience, health, and well-being in people, groups, and societies worldwide if responsible practices are upheld.

CHAPTER IX

Future Directions in Herbal Antiviral Research and Practice

Emerging Trends and Innovations

The field of natural healing is changing due to new developments and trends in herbal medicine, which present new avenues for utilizing the therapeutic properties of medicinal plants to treat viral infections and enhance general health and wellness. Practitioners, academics, and entrepreneurs are investigating new methods, technologies, and apps to improve the effectiveness, security, and accessibility of herbal medicines as interest in herbal medicine grows and scientific research progresses. Novel and exciting approaches to harness the antiviral powers of nature could be made possible by emerging trends and breakthroughs, which have the potential to revolutionize the area of herbal medicine.

Creating innovative extraction and formulation strategies that maximize the bioavailability, stability, and effectiveness of herbal treatments is one developing trend in herbal medicine. To improve the concentration and absorption of bioactive components from medicinal plants, cutting-edge techniques like supercritical fluid extraction, ultrasonic extraction, and nanoencapsulation are added to traditional extraction procedures, including decoction, infusion, and maceration. These cutting-edge extraction techniques enable the creation of highly standardized, bioavailable, and concentrated herbal extracts that are simple to combine into a range of dosage forms, such as tinctures, pills, capsules, and topical treatments. Using cutting-edge extraction technology, herbal medicine practitioners may fully utilize the therapeutic potential of medicinal plants and build personalized formulations for specific health conditions, such as viral infections.

Furthermore, customized herbal therapy is becoming increasingly popular as a viable method of adjusting herbal treatments to specific requirements, inclinations, and health objectives. Practitioners can now evaluate genetic variations, metabolic profiles, and health data to establish tailored treatment strategies and optimize herbal formulations for individual patients thanks to genomics, metabolomics, and personalized medicine advancements. To tailor herbal medicines based on genetic predispositions, biochemical markers, and environmental factors, personalized herbal medicine may involve genetic testing, diagnostic evaluations, and lifestyle changes. Herbal medicine practitioners can treat patients more effectively and precisely, improve patient outcomes, and raise the standard of care by adopting a tailored approach.

Moreover, online platforms and digital technology are transforming the availability, practice, and distribution of herbal medicine, increasing the accessibility and convenience of herbal medicines for people all over the world. Consumers may easily explore herbs, access instructional materials, and buy herbal cures thanks to the abundance of information, tools, and goods available on mobile applications, websites, and e-commerce platforms dedicated to herbal medicine. Patients can contact herbal medicine practitioners virtually and through telemedicine to receive individualized advice and access herbal medicines from the comfort of their own homes. Furthermore, wearable technology and digital health tracking tools enable people to track their progress, monitor their health data, and incorporate herbal medicines into their regular wellness routines.

Herbal medicine practitioners can increase patient involvement, collaborate and communicate more within the herbal medicine community, and reach a wider audience using digital technology.

Furthermore, new information on the antiviral characteristics and modes of action of medicinal plants is being revealed by scientific studies and clinical trials, offering essential insights into their possible use in diagnosing, treating, and preventing viral infections. Scholars are examining the effectiveness of particular herbs and botanical chemicals in combating various viruses, including influenza, herpes, HIV, and coronaviruses, as well as delving into the molecular mechanisms underlying their actions. To provide evidence-based recommendations and regulatory approvals, preclinical and clinical research assesses the antiviral effectiveness, safety, and pharmacokinetics of herbal medicines in human and animal models. Furthermore, cooperative research initiatives, including scientists, healthcare practitioners, and traditional healers, strengthen the connection between traditional knowledge and contemporary science, expanding our comprehension of herbal therapy and its possible uses in treating infectious diseases.

Furthermore, as awareness of environmental preservation, social responsibility, and cultural preservation grows, the herbal medicine sector is paying more and more attention to ethical harvesting methods and sustainable sourcing. To avoid overharvesting, habitat destruction, and biodiversity loss, there is an increasing need to guarantee the sustainability and ethical sourcing of botanical resources in response to the rising demand for medicinal plants. Sustainable harvesting practices are being promoted, local economies are being supported, and indigenous groups are empowered to conserve their traditional knowledge and cultural legacy through initiatives including community-based conservation programs, fair trade certification, and wildcrafting rules. Herbal medicine practitioners and stakeholders may support the long-term resilience and health of ecosystems and communities while guaranteeing the availability and accessibility of medicinal plants for future generations by prioritizing sustainability and ethical sourcing.

In conclusion, discoveries in the natural healing field are fueled by trends and innovations in herbal medicine, which present fresh chances to harness the antiviral properties of medicinal plants and advance well-being. Digital technology, tailored treatments, sophisticated extraction techniques, sustainable sourcing methods, and other developing trends and breakthroughs can completely transform the study, practice, and availability of herbal medicine. Herbal medicine practitioners may empower people to use the healing powers of nature in novel and transformative ways and improve the efficacy, safety, and accessibility of herbal treatments by embracing these trends and developments.

Potential Challenges and Opportunities

To optimize the advantages of herbal therapy in preventing viral infections and advancing public health, it is necessary to skillfully traverse the opportunities and possible difficulties of harnessing herbs' antiviral properties. Herbal treatments present a promising path for treatment and prevention but have limitations. These include cultural preconceptions, quality control issues, regulatory obstacles, and sustainability concerns. However, by taking proactive measures to overcome these issues and seizing new opportunities, interested parties can fully utilize herbal antivirals and open the door to a more comprehensive and integrated approach to managing infectious diseases.

The need for solid scientific data and established protocols to support the safety and efficacy of herbal antiviral medicines is one of their main problems. Herbal medical methods have traditionally been guided by anecdotal evidence and traditional knowledge. However, more and more comprehensive scientific studies and clinical trials are needed to validate the protective effects of botanical compounds and herbs against viral infections. Clinical research is crucial to clarify the pharmacokinetics, ideal dosage schedules, and mechanisms of action of herbal antivirals and spot possible drug interactions. Standardized procedures and quality control methods are also required to guarantee the potency, consistency, and purity of herbal products and reduce the possibility of contamination, adulteration, or mislabeling.

Furthermore, the development, marketing, and distribution of herbal antiviral treatments are significantly impeded by regulatory constraints. Countries differ greatly in their regulatory frameworks for herbal goods; sometimes, there must be clear regulations or supervision mechanisms to license, register, and label herbal treatments. The market may become confusing and inconsistent due to this lack of harmonization, making it more difficult for customers to obtain secure and efficient herbal medications. Furthermore, manufacturers of herbal medicines—especially small-scale producers and traditional healers—may find it expensive and time-consuming to comply with regulatory standards for clinical trials, product testing, and labeling. To establish a conducive atmosphere for the creation and application of herbal antiviral treatments, it is imperative to simplify regulatory procedures and encourage global cooperation and harmonization initiatives.

Moreover, maintaining the safety and effectiveness of herbal antiviral medications presents significant hurdles in quality control and assurance. The purity and therapeutic efficacy of herbal medicines can be compromised by problems like adulteration, substitution, and contamination, which pose a risk to the herbal medicine industry. During cultivation, harvesting, processing, or storage, herbal products may become polluted with pesticides, heavy metals, or microbiological infections, which could harm the end user's health. Furthermore, the public's belief in herbal treatment may be weakened by the abundance of fake or inferior herbal goods on the market. Maintaining quality standards and safeguarding customer safety requires vigorous quality control systems, such as third-party certification programs, sound manufacturing and farming practices, and standardized testing techniques.

Despite these difficulties, using herbs' antiviral properties also offers many chances for creativity, empowerment, and teamwork. Flavonoids, polyphenols, alkaloids, and essential oils are just a few of the bioactive substances in herbal medicine that have broad-spectrum antiviral qualities. Additionally, these substances have the power to boost host defense mechanisms, impede virus replication, and alter immune responses. By examining the antiviral properties of medicinal plants and identifying herbal combinations that work well together, researchers can develop novel formulations and medicines for the prevention and treatment of viral infections. By integrating herbal medicine into traditional healthcare systems and promoting interdisciplinary collaboration between traditional healers, scientists, and healthcare professionals, we can advance our understanding of herbal antivirals and enable greater access to safe and effective treatments.

In addition, growing interest in herbal medicine is fueled by consumer demand for all-natural, holistic approaches to health and well-being, opening up new avenues for market expansion. The demand for dietary supplements, herbal medicines, and antiviral products is rising as consumers look for alternatives to prescription drugs and adopt preventative healthcare practices. The need for safe, efficient, scientifically supported herbal medicines is growing, which presents opportunities for practitioners, manufacturers, and merchants. Consumers increasingly use herbal medicine for immune support, symptom alleviation, and general well-being. Furthermore, digital technologies and online platforms provide new channels for outreach, education, and cooperation within the herbal medicine community. This allows practitioners to disseminate best practices, resources, and expertise to a worldwide audience.

Additionally, encouraging sustainability and moral sourcing in the herbal medicine sector offers chances to safeguard local economies, conserve traditional knowledge, and conserve cultural heritage while protecting biodiversity. To guarantee the long-term sustainability of medicinal plants and encourage environmental care, stakeholders should prioritize sustainable production, wildcrafting regulations, and fair trading standards. In addition, local communities can be empowered to manage their natural resources sustainably and reap the financial benefits of herbal medicine through community-based projects and partnerships between indigenous peoples, herbalists, and conservation organizations.

In summary, harnessing the potential of herbal remedies to combat viral infections has certain obstacles and prospects that call for cooperation, creativity, and conscientious management. Stakeholders may fully realize the promise of herbal medicine in preventing viral infections and advancing public health by removing regulatory obstacles, improving quality control procedures, encouraging scientific research, and embracing sustainability. With a focused effort to address these problems and seize new opportunities, herbal medicine has the potential to have a substantial impact on the management of infectious diseases in the future and to encourage a more integrated and balanced approach to health and wellness.

The Role of Herbal Medicine in Global Health Preparedness

Herbal medicine's place in global health preparedness is becoming more widely acknowledged as a valuable and complementary strategy to traditional healthcare systems, especially during pandemics and infectious disease outbreaks. Utilizing a wealth of botanical resources, traditional knowledge, and therapeutic approaches, herbal therapy can improve immunity, boost resilience, and lessen the harmful effects of viral infections on public health. Herbal medicine has a varied role in global health preparation, offering a holistic and integrative approach to addressing the complex issues of managing infectious diseases. These challenges range from symptom management and recovery to immune support and preventive methods.

Herbal medicine places a strong focus on immune support and preventative healthcare, which is one of its main contributions to global health preparedness. Bioactive substances found in high concentrations in herbal treatments, such as vitamins, minerals, antioxidants, and phytochemicals, have been demonstrated to influence host defense systems, adjust immunological responses, and improve general health. Immune-strengthening herbs and botanical supplements can be a daily part of health routines that help people become less susceptible to illnesses and more resilient to environmental stressors.

Traditional methods, including herbal teas, tonics, and nutritional supplements that support respiratory health, encourage detoxification, and preserve immunological balance, are also provided by herbal medicine. These methods help to stop the spread of infectious diseases and lessen their adverse effects on the world's health.

Herbal medicine is also essential for managing symptoms and providing supportive care during pandemics and virus outbreaks. A wide range of antiviral, anti-inflammatory, and immunomodulatory qualities found in herbal treatments can help reduce symptoms like fever, cough, congestion, and exhaustion, enhancing patient comfort and quality of life. Herbal tinctures, syrups, and capsules give focused support for immune function, stress reduction, and symptom alleviation; herbal teas, steam inhalations, and herbal poultices offer natural treatment for respiratory symptoms and encourage expectoration. Medical practitioners can offer patients comprehensive, personalized care that considers their physical, emotional, and spiritual needs while they recover from illness by integrating herbal medicine into conventional healthcare systems.

Additionally, by encouraging community resilience, self-reliance, and empowerment in the face of health emergencies, herbal medicine advances global health preparation. To empower people to take control of their health and well-being, traditional healers, herbalists, and community health workers play a crucial role in sharing information, tools, and valuable skills for using herbal medicine within their communities. Access to locally grown herbs and botanical cures is made possible by community-based projects like herbal gardens, apothecaries, and wellness centers, which promote resilience and self-sufficiency during difficult times.

Furthermore, customary medical procedures and cultural ceremonies provide consolation, encouragement, and a feeling of community during trying times, enhancing social cohesiveness and group resilience in the face of hardship.

Additionally, by encouraging ecological sustainability, biodiversity conservation, and environmental stewardship, herbal medicine aids in the preparation of the world's health. A large number of medicinal plants are taken from natural environments, where they are essential to preserving biodiversity, ecological resilience, and ecosystem balance. The long-term survival of medicinal plants is ensured by sustainable cultivation, ethical harvesting methods, and wildcrafting principles, promoting the well-being of the ecosystems and communities that depend on them. Herbal medicine practitioners and stakeholders may safeguard biodiversity, maintain traditional knowledge, and lessen the ecological effects of global health crises by encouraging sustainable sourcing and conservation of medicinal plants.

Herbal medicine also encourages multidisciplinary study, teamwork, and creativity in the realm of managing infectious diseases. Researchers, scientists, and medical professionals are devoting more and more time to studying the therapeutic potential, mechanisms of action, and antiviral qualities of medicinal plants and botanical chemicals in the prevention and treatment of viral infections. Research on the pharmacokinetics, safety, and effectiveness of herbal treatments against various viruses, including coronaviruses, influenza, and newly developing infectious illnesses, is being conducted in preclinical and clinical settings. Our understanding of herbal medicine and its role in global health preparation is enhanced by collaborative research efforts involving scientists, public health specialists, and traditional healers that bridge the gap between traditional knowledge and modern science.

In summary, herbal medicine is dynamic and diverse regarding community resilience, preventative medicine, supportive care, ecological sustainability, and scientific innovation, all essential aspects of global health preparation. Stakeholders can fully utilize herbal medicine to improve health equity, boost resilience, and lessen the effects of pandemics and infectious disease outbreaks on the world's population by integrating it into traditional healthcare systems, encouraging sustainable practices, empowering communities, and fostering interdisciplinary collaboration. Herbal medicine can significantly contribute to enhancing global health readiness and creating a more resilient and sustainable future for all, provided that it is used with a deliberate effort to integrate traditional knowledge, scientific data, and community resources.

CHAPTER X

Herbal Medicine in Public Health Initiatives

Utilizing Herbal Medicine in Disease Prevention Campaigns

Promoting public health and battling infectious diseases may be accomplished through herbal medicine in disease preventive initiatives. Because of its ability to strengthen immunity and combat disease, herbal treatments have long been a part of traditional medical systems worldwide. Including herbal medicine in disease prevention programs is a method that is both accessible and comprehensive, enabling people to take control of their health and lessening the toll that illness takes on healthcare systems. Public health programs can boost immunity, improve resilience, and slow the spread of infectious diseases within communities by utilizing the preventative potential of herbal medicine.

Because herbal medicine supports immune function and strengthens the body's natural defenses, it is an essential tool in the fight against disease. Bioactive substances, including polyphenols, flavonoids, and polysaccharides, which are abundant in medicinal plants, have been demonstrated to influence immunological responses, boost the formation of antibodies, and impede the growth of viruses. Due to their immune-stimulating qualities, herbal treatments, including echinacea, elderberry, astragalus, and garlic, are frequently used and have been used traditionally to prevent respiratory infections, such as colds, the flu, and other viral disorders. Including these immune-stimulating herbs in illness-preventive programs can help fortify the immune system, lessen infection susceptibility, and increase resistance to viral infections in general.

Moreover, herbal therapy is a secure and economical method of illness prevention, especially in areas with low resources where access to traditional healthcare may be restricted. Herbal medicines can benefit a broad spectrum of people, including underprivileged and marginalized communities because they are frequently easily obtained, reasonably priced, and culturally acceptable. Regardless of socioeconomic level or geography, initiatives to prevent illness may encourage individuals to take control of their health and well-being through the promotion of locally grown medicinal plants and traditional herbal treatments. Herbal medicine also supports the ideas of self-care and empowerment by enticing people to embrace preventive measures to ward against infectious diseases and good lifestyle choices.

Incorporating herbal medicine into illness-prevention efforts by fostering traditional knowledge, cultural practices, and intergenerational learning promotes social cohesiveness and community resilience. Herbal medicine has a rich history in many cultures that has been passed down through the generations, offering essential insights into medicinal herbs' use for illness prevention and treatment. Disease prevention campaigns can access this wealth of information and experience by collaborating with local healers, practitioners of traditional medicine, and community leaders. This allows them to customize interventions to each community's unique requirements and cultural preferences. Furthermore, herbal gardens, seminars, and educational events are examples of community-based herbal medicine programs offering opportunities for skill development, knowledge exchange, and social interaction. These initiatives foster community links and encourage group health initiatives.

Additionally, herbal medicine offers a comprehensive and integrated strategy for improving health and wellness, supplementing traditional healthcare interventions in campaigns to avoid disease. As critical preventive measures against infectious diseases, such as vaccinations, drugs, and good hygiene, herbal medicines can also be used as supportive therapies to boost immunity, lessen the severity of symptoms, and promote general health. A multifaceted approach to disease prevention is made possible by integrating herbal medicine into comprehensive preventative methods, which target biological and psychosocial factors that influence health outcomes. Herbal medicine can also help close gaps in the current healthcare system by offering alternatives to people who might find it difficult to receive traditional treatments or would instead use natural, non-invasive methods to maintain their health.

In summary, integrating herbal medicine into disease-preventive initiatives presents a comprehensive, attainable, and culturally appropriate strategy for advancing public health and addressing infectious diseases. Public health programs can enhance immune function, empower individuals, promote community resilience, and supplement traditional healthcare interventions by utilizing the preventative potential of herbal therapies. Incorporating herbal medicine into disease prevention efforts improves the health of individuals and communities and advances the larger objective of social justice and health equity for all.

Herbal Medicine in Epidemic and Pandemic Response Strategies

Because herbal medicine provides a comprehensive and integrated strategy for managing infectious diseases and fostering public health resilience, it plays a vital role in epidemic and pandemic response plans. Herbal medicines are valuable for supportive care, symptom management, and prevention during epidemics and pandemics. They enhance general resilience to viral outbreaks and complement conventional healthcare measures. Herbal medicine helps to provide a comprehensive and multifaceted response to infectious disease emergencies by utilizing the antiviral qualities, immune-boosting effects, and traditional knowledge of medicinal plants. This empowers individuals, communities, and healthcare systems to reduce the impact on public health and minimize the spread of infection.

Herbal medicine is significant in immune support and preventive measures to react to epidemics and pandemics. Bioactive substances found in high concentrations in herbal treatments, such as flavonoids, alkaloids, and essential oils, have been demonstrated to influence host defense mechanisms, suppress viral replication, and modify immunological responses.

Immune-strengthening herbs and botanical supplements can be used in public health initiatives to help people become more resilient to viral pathogens, less prone to infection, and more robust against infection. Herbal medicine also provides traditional methods that support respiratory health, encourage detoxification, and maintain immune balance. These methods, along with herbal teas, tonics, and nutritional supplements, help to reduce the spread of infectious diseases and lessen their impact on public health.

Herbal medicine is also essential for managing symptoms and providing supportive care during pandemics and epidemics. Numerous medicinal plants include analgesic, antiviral, and anti-inflammatory qualities that can help reduce symptoms, including weariness, fever, coughing, and congestion, while also enhancing patient comfort and quality of life. Herbal treatments with anti-inflammatory and immune-modulating properties, like elderberry, licorice root, ginger, and turmeric, are frequently used to relieve respiratory symptoms naturally and aid in healing after viral infections. By incorporating herbal medicine into traditional healthcare systems, medical professionals may provide patients with all-encompassing, individualized care that considers their physical, emotional, and psychological requirements while they recover from disease.

Moreover, herbal medicine supports pandemic and epidemic response tactics by encouraging community resilience, self-reliance, and empowerment in the face of health emergencies. To empower people to take control of their health and well-being, traditional healers, herbalists, and community health workers play a crucial role in sharing information, tools, and valuable skills for using herbal medicine within their communities. Access to locally grown herbs and botanical cures is made possible by community-based projects like herbal gardens, apothecaries, and wellness centers, which promote resilience and self-sufficiency during difficult times.

Furthermore, customary medical procedures and cultural ceremonies provide consolation, encouragement, and a feeling of community during trying times, enhancing social cohesiveness and group resilience in the face of hardship.

Additionally, incorporating herbal medicine into pandemic and epidemic response plans encourages cooperation and ingenuity in healthcare provision. Researchers, scientists, and medical professionals are devoting more and more time to studying the therapeutic potential, mechanisms of action, and antiviral qualities of medicinal plants and botanical chemicals in preventing and treating viral infections. Research on the pharmacokinetics, safety, and effectiveness of herbal treatments against various viruses, including coronaviruses, influenza, and newly developing infectious illnesses, is being conducted in preclinical and clinical settings. To close the knowledge gap between traditional healers and modern science, traditional healers, scientists, and public health specialists collaborate on research projects that deepen our understanding of herbal therapy and its application to pandemic and epidemic preparedness.

In summary, herbal medicine provides a comprehensive, approachable, and culturally appropriate means of managing infectious diseases and fostering public health resilience, making it an essential component of epidemic and pandemic response plans. Herbal remedies support a comprehensive and multifaceted response to viral outbreaks by utilizing antiviral qualities, immune-boosting effects, and traditional knowledge of medicinal plants. This empowers individuals, communities, and healthcare systems to reduce the impact on public health and mitigate the spread of infection. Incorporating herbal medicine into traditional healthcare systems encourages teamwork, creativity, and adaptability, advancing social justice and health equity for all.

Community-Based Herbal Medicine Programs for Underserved Populations

Programs for community-based herbal medicine embody a comprehensive strategy for providing healthcare that prioritizes addressing the needs of marginalized communities. Through herbal remedies and traditional medical practices, these initiatives are essential in addressing health inequities, improving well-being, and empowering communities. Millions lack access to primary medical treatment because conventional healthcare services are restricted or impossible to obtain in many parts of the world, especially in low-income and rural communities. Programs for community-based herbal medicine close this gap by providing readily available, reasonably priced, culturally aware healthcare options that emphasize community involvement, education, and prevention.

One of its main advantages is the focus on preventative healthcare that community-based herbal medicine programs place. These initiatives give proactive approaches to preserving health and preventing disease priority above only treating illnesses once they arise. Herbal medicines fortify the body's natural defenses and enhance general wellness. They are frequently abundant in nutrients and immune-boosting substances. Community-based initiatives give people the tools to take charge of their health and well-being by teaching them about herbal medicine and self-care techniques. This will eventually improve health outcomes and lower healthcare expenditures.

Additionally, community-based herbal medicine initiatives are designed to accommodate marginalized communities' particular requirements and inclinations. In many cultures, herbal cures and traditional healing methods have solid cultural roots passed down through the years as a cultural legacy and identity component. Community-based programs ensure that healthcare interventions are relevant and sensitive to cultural differences by honoring and respecting these traditions and establishing rapport and trust with community members. To provide treatment, offer culturally sensitive services, and close the knowledge gap between conventional medicine and contemporary healthcare systems, herbalists, traditional healers, and community health workers frequently play crucial roles.

Furthermore, community-based herbal medicine initiatives support marginalized communities' self-determination and empowerment. These initiatives enable people, regardless of socioeconomic class or geographic location, to take charge of their health and well-being by teaching them how to cultivate, collect, and prepare medicinal plants. Herbal medicine gardens, communal herb walks, and interactive workshops offer chances for social interaction, knowledge exchange, and skill development, enhancing community links and encouraging group health initiatives. In addition, community-based initiatives often integrate advocacy, community organizing, and leadership training components, enabling people to speak up for their health needs and organize for social change.

Furthermore, community-based herbal medicine programs support health equity by addressing social determinants of health and facilitating access to culturally competent care. Financial limitations, transportation issues, and language hurdles are just a few of the obstacles that many marginalized communities must overcome to receive traditional healthcare services. Community-based programs get over these obstacles by providing healthcare services directly to the public—typically through outreach programs, mobile clinics, and community health centers. These programs guarantee that all individuals have access to the necessary resources for achieving maximum health and well-being by meeting people where they are and offering treatment in comfortable and dependable environments.

In summary, community-based herbal medicine initiatives are crucial for campaigns to advance health justice and enhance results for marginalized groups. These programs provide holistic answers to healthcare problems by emphasizing prevention, empowerment, and community involvement. They also use herbal treatments and traditional healing methods to address the underlying causes of sickness and advance well-being. As we work to develop more inclusive and equitable healthcare systems, community-based herbal medicine programs guarantee that everyone has access to the tools they need to thrive and act as role models for grassroots creativity, social justice, and community resilience.

CHAPTER XI

Ethical Considerations and Cultural Competence in Herbal Medicine

Practice Respecting Cultural Traditions and Indigenous Knowledge

Herbal medicine requires respect for indigenous knowledge and cultural customs, especially when using herbs with antiviral properties. Indigenous cultures worldwide have created sophisticated traditional medicine systems over many generations because they have a close understanding of the local flora, ecosystems, and healing methods. These practices are essential to indigenous peoples' identity and legacy, rooted in social mores, spirituality, and cultural beliefs. Herbalists and medical professionals must approach traditional medicine systems with humility, respect, and an openness to gaining knowledge from indigenous populations.

Recognizing the experience and authority of indigenous healers and knowledge bearers is fundamental to respecting cultural traditions and indigenous knowledge. The expertise of traditional healers, sometimes referred to as shamans, medicine men, or herbalists, concerning medicinal plants, healing practices, and customary cures has been passed down through the years. Rather than having had formal academic training, their expertise is based on firsthand experience, observation, and oral transmission. Herbal medicine practitioners can foster reciprocal learning and exchange, form meaningful partnerships, and foster trust by acknowledging and appreciating the expertise and wisdom of indigenous healers.

Furthermore, appreciating indigenous knowledge and cultural traditions necessitates comprehending and valuing medicinal herbs' spiritual and cultural importance to indigenous people. Plants are considered sacred creatures in many traditional cultures, possessing inherent healing and spiritual abilities. Rituals, prayers, and sacrifices are frequently used in traditional healing ceremonies, rituals, and practices to call upon the spiritual powers of plants and foster a connection with the natural world. Herbalists can develop a deeper appreciation for the interconnection of all living things and a deeper grasp of the spiritual aspects of herbal medicine by reverently and respectfully participating in these ceremonies.

Additionally, using medicinal plants and traditional treatments demands ethical and responsible behavior to respect indigenous knowledge and cultural traditions. This entails respecting intellectual property rights, getting the informed agreement of indigenous groups before using their knowledge and resources, and fairly dividing the advantages. Instead of being founded on exploitation or appropriation, cooperation and partnerships with indigenous groups should be founded on the values of reciprocity, trust, and respect. Herbal medicine practitioners should also work to safeguard indigenous knowledge systems and traditional therapeutic methods because they have inherent value and contribute to the health and well-being of the world.

In addition, acknowledging and redressing past and present injustices against indigenous peoples—such as colonization, land theft, and cultural genocide—is essential to upholding indigenous knowledge and cultural practices. Indigenous knowledge has been lost, traditional healing methods have deteriorated, and indigenous lands and resources have been exploited for financial gain as a result of colonialism and globalization. Health disparities and socioeconomic inequality are exacerbated when indigenous people encounter institutional obstacles that limit their access to healthcare, education, and economic possibilities. Herbal medicine practitioners must uphold indigenous rights, back initiatives led by indigenous peoples for cultural revival and land sovereignty, and give voice to indigenous viewpoints in the herbal medicine community.

In conclusion, ethical and responsible herbal medicine practice requires respect for indigenous knowledge and cultural traditions. Herbal medicine practitioners can support the preservation, revitalization, and empowerment of indigenous communities by respecting the knowledge and experience of indigenous healers, honoring the spiritual and cultural significance of medicinal plants, practicing ethical and responsible behavior, and speaking up for the rights of indigenous people. Approaching this study with humility, respect, and dedication to social justice and cultural diversity is crucial as we harness the antiviral properties of herbs and investigate the possibilities of traditional medicine systems.

Addressing Ethical Dilemmas in Herbal Medicine Research and Practice

Previously confined to the periphery of medicine, herbal medicine is currently enjoying a renaissance in awareness and acceptance, especially when fighting viral infections. With the world struggling to contain viral outbreaks, such as the current COVID-19 pandemic, there is increased curiosity about the possible antiviral properties of herbal therapies. Notwithstanding this zeal, it is imperative to confront the moral problems that arise in the study and application of herbal medicine to guarantee the responsible and fair application of these treatments.

The regulation and standardization of herbal products are fundamental ethical concerns in herbal medicine. Standardized production procedures and quality control measures are typically absent from herbal treatments, in contrast to pharmaceutical pharmaceuticals subjected to stringent regulation and testing. This fluctuation casts doubt on herbal remedies' stability, safety, and potency, putting consumers at risk and making study findings more difficult to interpret. Promoting enhanced regulation and quality assurance methods is imperative for ethical practitioners and researchers to protect public health and bolster the legitimacy of herbal medicine.

Furthermore, informed permission and patient autonomy provide ethical obstacles to research on herbal therapy. Participants in clinical trials and research incorporating herbal interventions must receive sufficient information regarding the possible dangers, advantages, and uncertainties related to herbal treatments. However, getting fully informed permission might be difficult because of the complexity of herbal medicines and the lack of more available scientific data. Individuals may have erroneous or inadequate perceptions about herbal remedies due to cultural convictions, promotional assertions, or firsthand accounts. Transparently navigating these difficulties requires researchers and healthcare practitioners to respect patients' autonomy and choices while enabling them to make educated health decisions.

Incorporating herbal medicine into traditional healthcare systems also presents moral conundrums regarding responsibility and professional standards. Even though many healthcare professionals are aware of the potential benefits of herbal medications, the requirement for standardized education and training in herbal medicine poses issues in ensuring competency and ethical practice. Inadequate regulation and supervision may lead to incorrect prescribing methods, harmful interactions with traditional therapies, and misinformation. Professional standards and ethical guidelines should be established to ensure the proper integration of herbal medicine into clinical practice. These should prioritize continual education, interdisciplinary collaboration, and evidence-based approaches.

The ethical quandaries surrounding herbal medicine also encompass cultural appropriation and traditional knowledge exploitation. Traditional medical systems and indigenous practices are the origin of many herbal treatments. The intellectual property of indigenous people may be commercialized and profited from without due recognition or recompense if these cures become more and more popular in mainstream markets. In addition to upholding historical injustices, these practices also jeopardize indigenous peoples' autonomy and sovereignty over their traditional knowledge and resources. To guarantee indigenous people's involvement, permission, and benefit-sharing in herbal medicine research and commercialization initiatives, researchers and practitioners must engage in courteous engagement and communication with these populations.

Furthermore, research on herbal medicine encounters moral problems about commercialization and intellectual property rights as researchers delve into the medicinal qualities of plant-based chemicals and create innovative mixtures—concerns regarding property rights, patents, and profit-sharing schemes surface. The prioritization of financial gain over public health concerns in pursuing commercial interests may result in the monopolization of herbal knowledge and products. Prioritizing fair access to herbal resources, encouraging cooperation between the public and private sectors, and ensuring that herbal medicine research's advantages are distributed relatively among stakeholders—researchers, communities, and consumers—are all essential aspects of ethical frameworks.

In conclusion, it is critical to confront moral conundrums in herbal medicine research and practice to advance ethical, egalitarian, and long-term approaches to healthcare—especially when utilizing herbs' antiviral properties. Ethical issues are present in all facets of herbal therapy, from informed consent and cultural appropriation to regulation and standardization. Researchers, practitioners, policymakers, and communities can manage these difficulties while preserving the values of honesty, respect, and justice by thoughtfully discussing issues, working together, and making ethical decisions. In the end, the moral use of herbal medicine necessitates a dedication to openness, responsibility, and the welfare of people and society at large.

Promoting Cultural Competence and Diversity in Herbal Medicine Education

In the field of herbal medicine, in particular, the importance of cultural competence and diversity has emerged in recent years. Herbal medicine education programs must welcome cultural diversity and give students the knowledge and abilities to deliver culturally competent treatment as the demand for herbal therapies grows. Practitioners can better serve various patient communities, increase patient satisfaction and trust, and contribute to more equitable healthcare outcomes by encouraging cultural competence in herbal medicine education.

An essential component of fostering cultural competence in teaching herbal medicine is recognizing the wide range of therapeutic customs and methods that exist worldwide. Numerous indigenous and cultural traditions, each with distinct viewpoints, knowledge systems, and therapeutic techniques, are the deep roots of herbal medicine. A herbal medicine curriculum incorporating teachings from various cultural traditions helps students obtain a greater appreciation for the variety of healing modalities available and a broader awareness of the cultural context of herbal practice.

Promoting respect for cultural beliefs, values, and wellness-related activities is another way to advance cultural competency in herbal medicine teaching. Pupils need to identify and understand the cultural value that various communities place on herbs and medicinal practices—knowing how spiritual, ceremonial, and natural connections are part of customary healing methods. Herbal medicine students can develop trustworthy connections with patients from various backgrounds and deliver courteous, sensitive, and customized care to each patient's unique cultural preferences and needs by practicing cultural humility and open-mindedness.

Herbal medicine education programs should prioritize addressing health disparities and injustices in healthcare access, as well as cultural sensitivity and understanding. Access to high-quality healthcare, including services related to herbal medicine, is impeded for many marginalized communities, such as indigenous peoples, ethnic minorities, and socioeconomically disadvantaged groups. Students can better understand the systemic inequalities that influence health outcomes and contribute to health inequities by investigating the social determinants of health and the underlying causes of health disparities. Programs teaching herbal medicine should give students the tools to fight for equality and social justice in healthcare, both in the workplace and society.

Incorporating experiential learning opportunities that introduce students to various cultural viewpoints and healing practices is also necessary to promote cultural competence in herbal medicine education. Internships or clinical rotations in community-based settings catering to ethnically varied populations are possible examples of this, where students can watch and take part in culturally appropriate therapeutic approaches. Furthermore, integrating case studies, guest lectures, and workshops conducted by professionals with diverse cultural backgrounds can enhance students' educational experiences and expand their comprehension of cultural variations in health-related beliefs, practices, and consequences.

To effectively promote cultural competency in teaching herbal medicine, it is also crucial to cultivate multidisciplinary collaboration and discourse among practitioners, instructors, and students from various backgrounds. Herbal medicine education programs can foster a dynamic learning environment that fosters cross-cultural understanding, mutual respect, and cooperative problem-solving by bringing together people with diverse viewpoints, knowledge, and life experiences. Students who engage in interdisciplinary collaboration are better equipped to negotiate the nuanced cultural aspects of clinical practice and function well in diverse healthcare teams.

Additionally, practitioners and students must continue self-reflection and learning to promote cultural competence in herbal medicine education. Examining one's cultural prejudices, presumptions, and privileges is one way to do this, as is actively looking for ways to increase one's cultural competency by being exposed to various viewpoints and experiences. Herbal medicine practitioners can enhance their capacity to deliver culturally sensitive care and support social justice and health equity by committing to cultural humility and self-awareness.

To sum up, herbal medicine education must promote cultural competence and diversity to adequately prepare practitioners to serve a variety of communities and handle the complicated health demands of multicultural cultures.

Herbal medicine education programs can enable students to become culturally competent practitioners who contribute to more inclusive and equitable healthcare systems by incorporating teachings from diverse cultural traditions, fostering respect for cultural beliefs and practices, addressing health disparities, offering opportunities for experiential learning, facilitating interdisciplinary collaboration, and encouraging ongoing self-reflection and learning. In the end, encouraging cultural competence in teaching herbal medicine is a moral obligation and a vital tactic for advancing social justice in the healthcare industry, enhancing patient outcomes, and advancing health equity.

CHAPTER XII

Herbal Medicine and Mental Health

Herbal Remedies for Stress Reduction and Mental Well-Being

Stress is becoming a common problem that affects people's mental health and general well-being in today's fast-paced and demanding society. Herbal therapies provide a natural, holistic alternative to traditional treatments for stress management, even though there are other methods, such as medication, therapy, and lifestyle changes. Traditional medical systems have long used herbal medicine, with many plants valued for their adaptogenic qualities—their capacity to support balance and assist the body in adjusting to stress. Herbal treatments can be incorporated into stress-reduction plans to give people valuable tools for improving resilience and mental health.

Ashwagandha, or Withania somnifera, is a well-known herb for reducing stress. It has been used for millennia in Ayurvedic medicine as an adaptogen. It has been demonstrated that ashwagandha increases resilience to stress and lowers cortisol levels, the primary hormone associated with stress. Ashwagandha has been shown in studies to boost the body's stress response system and modulate neurotransmitter levels in the brain, which may help reduce feelings of anxiety and depression. Moreover, ashwagandha contains antioxidant qualities that might guard against oxidative stress, a factor linked to the emergence of mental health issues.

Another herb, Rhodiola rosea, or golden or Arctic root, has anti-stress solid qualities. In traditional medical systems, rhodiola has been used to treat exhaustion, improve cognitive function, and increase resilience to stress, especially in Scandinavia and Russia. Rhodiola has been linked to reduced cortisol levels and increased activity of neurotransmitters essential for mood regulation, like dopamine and serotonin, which may help control the body's stress response. Moreover, Rhodiola demonstrates adaptogenic qualities, which improve the body's ability to handle mental and physical stress.

Additionally, herbal teas' relaxing properties, such as Melissa Officinalis lemon balm and Matricaria chamomilla's chamomile, can encourage rest and lessen tension and anxiety. Mainly, apigenin, a chemical found in chamomile tea, binds to brain receptors to provide sedative and anxiolytic effects. Conversely, substances found in lemon balm, such as flavonoids and rosmarinic acid, have been demonstrated to lower cortisol levels and enhance mood. Including these herbal teas in everyday activities can create a calming ritual that supports stress relief and mental health.

Furthermore, it has long been known that adaptogenic herbs like Siberian ginseng (Eleutherococcus senticosus) and holy basil (Ocimum sanctum) strengthen the body's reaction to stress and foster resilience and mental clarity.

Ayurvedic medicine places excellent significance on tulsi, often known as holy basil, for its adaptogenic and anti-anxiety properties. Holy basil may help control cortisol levels, lessen depressive and anxious symptoms, and enhance cognitive performance, according to research. Likewise, research has demonstrated that Siberian ginseng, a well-liked adaptogen in traditional Chinese medicine, supports adrenal function, elevates mood, and improves mental and physical performance under stress.

Herbal blends containing several nervines and adaptogens and individual herbs can have synergistic benefits for lowering stress and promoting mental health. Herbal blends that combine ashwagandha, holy basil, rhodiola, and other stress-reducing herbs, for instance, can offer complete support for the body's stress response system, assisting people in managing everyday stressors and fostering emotional equilibrium. These formulations are easily accessible and convenient stress-reduction solutions because they are frequently offered in various formats, such as capsules, tinctures, and teas.

Moreover, deep breathing exercises, yoga, and meditation are mindfulness practices that might improve the efficiency of herbal medicines for stress relief. In addition to enhancing the benefits of herbal therapies, mindfulness practices assist people in developing present-moment awareness, minimizing rumination, and fostering calm. People can construct a comprehensive approach to stress management that treats both the physiological and psychological elements of stress by combining mindfulness activities with herbal treatments.

In conclusion, herbal medicines are beneficial for mental health and stress relief, offering all-natural substitutes for pharmaceutical treatments. Herbs that promote relaxation and emotional equilibrium, such as nervines like chamomile and lemon balm, also have calming properties that help the body adjust to stress and become more resilient. Examples of these herbs are ashwagandha, rhodiola, holy basil, and Siberian ginseng. Herbal medicines can help people reduce stress and create better resilience. Combined with mindfulness activities, they can also improve mental health and overall quality of life. To guarantee safety and efficacy, speaking with a trained healthcare provider before beginning any herbal regimen is crucial, mainly if you are on medication or have pre-existing medical conditions.

Herbal Approaches to Anxiety and Depression Management

Among the most common mental health conditions in the world, anxiety and depression affect millions of people and have a significant negative influence on quality of life. Herbal medicine provides an alternative strategy that is becoming more and more well-known for its efficacy and minimal risk of side effects, even while traditional treatments like psychotherapy and medication play a crucial part in controlling these diseases. Herbal remedies are made from plants and contain bioactive components that operate pharmacologically on the body's neurochemical pathways. These actions aid in improving emotional well-being and reduce symptoms of depression and anxiety.

This flowering plant, native to Europe and Asia, is called Hypericum perforatum, or St. John's Wort, and it is one of the most researched herbs for treating anxiety and depression. Hypericin and hyperforin, two bioactive substances found in St. John's wort, have been demonstrated to block the reuptake of neurotransmitters involved in mood modulation, including serotonin, dopamine, and norepinephrine. Studies suggest that for treating mild to severe depression, the medication St. John's Wort may be similarly beneficial as the antidepressant drug family known as selective serotonin reuptake inhibitors, or SSRIs. Clinical investigations have confirmed this.

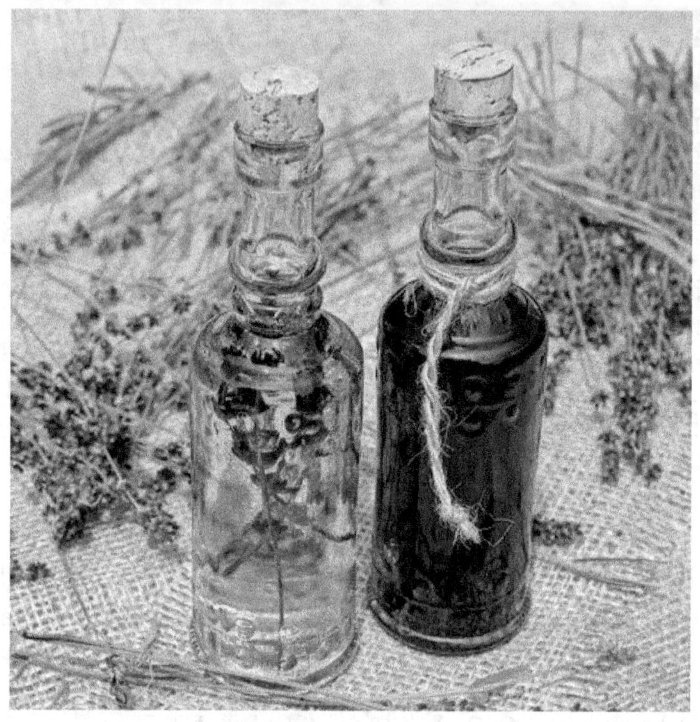

Lavender is another herb frequently used in herbal remedies for depression and anxiety (Lavandula angustifolia). Research has demonstrated that lavender essential oil, derived from the blossoms of the lavender plant, can reduce anxiety and promote emotional stability. Clinical studies have linked the inhalation or topical application of lavender oil to decreased anxiety, better sleep, and elevated mood. The capacity of lavender to alter the action of gamma-aminobutyric acid (GABA), a neurotransmitter that encourages relaxation and lowers excitability in the central nervous system, is thought to be the mechanism underlying the soothing effects of lavender.

Moreover, ashwagandha, or Withania somnifera, is an adaptogenic plant that has demonstrated potential in the treatment of anxiety and depression. Withanolides, a class of bioactive chemicals found in ashwagandha, modulate neurotransmitter levels, reduce inflammation, and enhance adrenal function to produce anxiolytic and antidepressant effects. Supplementing with ashwagandha may lessen the symptoms of anxiety and depression, increase stress tolerance, and improve general well- being, according to research. Moreover, those who are under prolonged stress, which frequently contributes to anxiety and depression, can benefit significantly from ashwagandha's adaptogenic qualities.

Another herbal treatment used traditionally for its sedative and relaxing properties is passionflower (Passiflora incarnata). Flavonoids and alkaloids found in passionflower affect the central nervous system, promote relaxation, and lessen symptoms of anxiety and insomnia. Clinical studies have demonstrated the potential of passionflower supplements to lower anxiety levels and enhance the quality of sleep, making them a proper herbal remedy for those with anxiety-related sleep disorders. Passionflower is also suitable for long-term use because it is generally well-tolerated and has a minimal risk of adverse effects.

Herbal formulations combining several anxiolytic and mood-stabilizing herbs, in addition to individual herbs, can have synergistic effects for managing anxiety and depression. Herbal mixtures, including St. John's Wort, lavender, ashwagandha, and passionflower, may offer all-encompassing assistance for mental health and stress tolerance. For all-natural alternatives to traditional therapies, these formulations are easily accessible and readily available in various forms, such as capsules, tinctures, and teas.

Moreover, a holistic approach to managing anxiety and depression must take into account lifestyle aspects like nutrition, exercise, and stress reduction methods. A balanced diet full of nutrient-dense foods, regular exercise, adequate sleep, and stress-reduction methods like mindfulness and meditation help enhance general mental health and well-being in addition to the benefits of herbal medications. People can enhance the effectiveness of herbal therapies and lower their chances of recurrence by combining specific lifestyle changes with them.

In conclusion, a rising body of research is demonstrating the efficacy and safety of herbal approaches to the management of anxiety and depression, making them attractive substitutes for traditional therapies. Herbs helpful in fostering emotional resilience and well-being include St. John's Wort, lavender, ashwagandha, and passionflower. These plants include bioactive chemicals with anxiolytic, mood-stabilizing, and stress-reducing properties. Before starting any herbal regimen, you should see an experienced physician to ensure that it is safe and effective, especially if you are using a prescription or have a history of medical issues. Herbal medications, lifestyle modifications, and other holistic approaches can help people take preventative action to manage their depression and anxiety and reach optimal mental health. See a licensed healthcare professional before beginning any herbal regimen to ensure safety and efficacy, particularly if you are taking prescription medication or have a medical history. Herbal medications, lifestyle modifications, and other holistic approaches can help people take preventative action to manage their depression and anxiety and reach optimal mental health.

Integration of Herbal Medicine into Holistic Mental Health Care

A paradigm shift in how mental health illnesses are treated is represented by the incorporation of herbal medicine into holistic mental health care. Recognizing the connection between the mind, body, and spirit, holistic mental health treatment treats the patient as a whole, taking into account underlying imbalances and contributing causes in addition to symptoms. Herbal medicine is a supplementary method that tackles mental health from numerous aspects and promotes general well-being. It is in line with the ideas of holistic care, as it focuses on natural therapies derived from plant sources.

The emphasis on individualized treatment regimens catered to each patient's needs and preferences is one of the main benefits of using herbal medicine in holistic mental health care treatment. With the wide range of alternatives provided by herbal treatments, practitioners can tailor treatment plans to the individual's biochemistry, underlying imbalances, and the type and degree of symptoms. Rather than only using medications to cover up symptoms, practitioners can promote the body's natural healing ability and address the underlying causes of mental health illnesses by adopting a tailored strategy.

Furthermore, by treating underlying imbalances and dysfunctions that lead to psychological suffering in addition to the symptoms of mental illness, herbal medicine offers a comprehensive approach to mental health. Many herbs used in mental health care have adaptogenic qualities, which means they aid in the body's ability to adjust to stress and realign the neurological system. As an illustration, adaptogens such as holy basil, ashwagandha, and Rhodiola improve adrenal function, control cortisol levels, and alter neurotransmitter activity, all of which assist in lessening the symptoms of depression, anxiety, and other mood disorders.
In addition, the incorporation of herbal medicine into holistic mental health care underscores the significance of tackling lifestyle issues like nutrition, physical activity, rest, and stress reduction that affect mental health.

Herbal treatments can assist with these lifestyle changes and foster resilience and general health. Herbs with anti-inflammatory qualities that boost brain health and cognitive function include turmeric and ginger, while chamomile and passionflower can help induce relaxation and enhance the quality of sleep.

Herbal compositions, including several botanical substances, in addition to individual herbs, can have synergistic effects that support mental health. Herbal mixes that combine nervines, adaptogens, and mood-stabilizing herbs, for instance, may offer complete support for stress resilience and emotional well-being. These formulations, which are often designed to address specific mental health disorders like sorrow, anxiety, or mood swings, can be tailored to match the individual needs of each user through careful ingredient and dosage selection.

Furthermore, by giving people the means and resources to participate actively in their recovery process, integrating herbal medicine into holistic mental health care encourages patient empowerment and self-care. Compared to pharmaceutical drugs, herbal medicines are frequently more readily available, reasonably priced, and low-risk, which makes them appropriate for long-term usage and self-administration. Patients must experience agency and autonomy in order to recover from mental illness over the long term. This can be achieved by giving them the power to make decisions about their own health and well-being.

Herbalists, naturopathic doctors, psychiatrists, therapists, and other healthcare professionals collaborate and communicate across disciplines when herbal medicine is incorporated into holistic mental health treatment. To create complete treatment plans that meet the many requirements of people with mental health issues, practitioners can benefit from each other's distinct areas of expertise and views when they collaborate. By highlighting the value of dialogue, mutual respect, and collaborative decision-making, this integrated care paradigm eventually improves the caliber and efficacy of mental health services.

In conclusion, a potential strategy for treating the intricate and multidimensional nature of mental illness is the incorporation of herbal medicine into holistic mental health care. By emphasizing customized treatment plans, addressing underlying imbalances, promoting lifestyle adjustments, and fostering patient empowerment and participation, herbal medicine can be a valuable tool in improving mental health and well-being. It's crucial to understand, though, that herbal remedies are not a cure-all and might not be suitable for every person or every mental health issue. As with any treatment, it's critical to speak with a licensed healthcare professional to ascertain the best course of action based on unique requirements, preferences, and circumstances. Herbal medicine can be combined synergistically with other forms of care to promote holistic mental health and wellness, but this requires careful thought and well-informed decision-making.

CHAPTER XIII

Herbal Medicine and Chronic Disease Management

Herbal Therapies for Chronic Conditions such as Diabetes, Hypertension, and Autoimmune Disorders

Worldwide, people with chronic illnesses like diabetes, hypertension, and autoimmune disorders face enormous problems in accessing treatment. Herbal remedies provide a supplemental strategy to enhance general health and well-being, even if conventional medicines are frequently required to manage specific problems. With its focus on all-natural treatments derived from plants, herbal medicine offers a wide range of choices for treating the underlying imbalances and encouraging holistic healing in persistent illnesses.

Native to Asia, Africa, and the Caribbean, bitter melon (Momordica charantia) is a fruit-bearing plant extensively studied as a herbal remedy for long-term ailments, including diabetes. Bioactive components of bitter melon, including charantin, polypeptide-p, and vicine, have been shown to lower blood sugar and improve insulin sensitivity. Clinical research has shown that supplementing with bitter melon can effectively lower fasting blood glucose and HbA1c levels, making it a helpful adjuvant treatment for diabetics. Furthermore, bitter melon has anti-inflammatory and antioxidant qualities that may help lessen the effects of diabetes-related problems like neuropathy and cardiovascular disease.

Similar to this, patients with diabetes have traditionally utilized the plant's fenugreek (Trigonella foenum-graecum) and cinnamon (Cinnamomum verum) to help regulate their blood sugar levels and improve their sensitivity to insulin. It has been demonstrated that substances found in cinnamon, such as cinnamaldehyde and cinnamon mix acid, improve insulin signaling and glucose uptake in cells. Studies have shown that taking supplements containing cinnamon can help persons with type 2 diabetes improve their lipid profiles and reduce their fasting blood glucose levels. Similarly, fenugreek seeds are high in soluble fiber and bioactive substances like galactomannan and trigonelline, which aid in reducing postprandial blood sugar increases and slowing down the absorption of carbohydrates.

In addition, herbal remedies can be beneficial supplements to traditional medicine in the management of hypertension, which is a significant risk indicator for heart disease and stroke. Herbs that improve cardiovascular health and encourage good blood pressure levels include hibiscus (Hibiscus sabdariffa), garlic (Allium sativum), and hawthorn (Crataegus spp.). Flavonoids and oligomeric procyanidins found in hawthorn berries have vasodilatory actions and enhance blood flow to the heart muscle, lowering blood pressure and maintaining cardiac function. On the other hand, research has shown that the sulfur-containing chemicals in garlic, like allicin and diallyl sulfide, lower blood pressure by inhibiting the angiotensin-converting enzyme (ACE) and promoting vasodilation. Comparably, the antioxidants included in hibiscus tea, such as anthocyanins and polyphenols, aid to relax blood vessels and reduce blood pressure.

Additionally, those with autoimmune disorders—disorders in which the immune system incorrectly targets healthy tissues and organs—can benefit from herbal therapy. Herbs with anti-inflammatory and immunomodulatory qualities, such as licorice (Glycyrrhiza glabra), ginger (Zingiber officinale), and turmeric (Curcuma longa), can help control the immune system and lessen the symptoms of autoimmune diseases. The key ingredient in turmeric, curcumin, has been the subject of much research due to its potential to reduce inflammation and suppress the production of inflammatory cytokines and immune cell activation. Like other autoimmune illnesses, rheumatoid arthritis, multiple sclerosis, and other symptoms of inflammation may be lessened by the chemicals gingerol and shogaol found in ginger. Glycyrrhizin, a substance found in licorice root, has potent anti-inflammatory and immunomodulatory properties. It has been demonstrated to alleviate symptoms and lower disease activity in autoimmune diseases such as lupus and rheumatoid arthritis.

Herbal compositions, including several botanical compounds, as opposed to single herbs, can synergistically affect chronic ailments such as diabetes, hypertension, and autoimmune disorders. Herbal blends that combine blood sugar-regulating herbs like cinnamon, fenugreek, and bitter melon or cardiovascular-supporting herbs like hibiscus, hawthorn, and garlic can offer comprehensive assistance for controlling many illnesses. Similarly, herbal formulas that contain ingredients like turmeric, ginger, and licorice and are intended to control the immune system and reduce inflammation can provide comprehensive support for people suffering from autoimmune disorders.

In conclusion, long-term conditions, including diabetes, high blood pressure, and autoimmune diseases, can be effectively treated using herbal therapies. They can be used as supplements or natural substitutes for traditional medical interventions. Herbs can assist with addressing underlying imbalances, promoting optimal physiological functioning, and supporting general well-being due to their vast array of bioactive chemicals and action methods. To guarantee safety and efficacy, it is imperative that you speak with a trained healthcare provider before beginning any herbal regimen, mainly if you are on medication or have pre-existing medical conditions. People can improve their quality of life and maximize treatment results when managing chronic diseases by combining herbal therapy with other holistic techniques and lifestyle improvements.

Herbal Medicine in Integrative Cancer Care

Herbal medicine is a complementary and alternative modality used in integrative cancer care, a comprehensive approach to cancer treatment. Herbal medicine has long been used in supportive care and cancer therapy. Numerous herbs are highly valued for their potential anti-cancer, immune-boosting, and symptom-management advantages. Patients can access a wider choice of treatment options and receive all- encompassing support for their physical, mental, and spiritual well-being throughout their cancer journey by incorporating herbal medicine into their cancer care.

Immune system stimulation and the body's natural defenses are two of herbal medicine's primary functions in integrative cancer care. Numerous herbs have immune-modulating qualities that support immune surveillance against cancer cells and help control the immune response. Herbs that have been traditionally used to boost immunity and increase resistance to illnesses and sickness include echinacea (Echinacea purpurea), reishi mushroom (Ganoderma lucidum), and astragalus (Astragalus membranaceus). These herbs may help lower the chance of cancer recurrence and enhance the body's resistance to the adverse effects of traditional cancer therapies like radiation therapy and chemotherapy by boosting immune function.

Additionally, herbal therapy can help cancer patients live better lives by reducing the negative consequences of their treatment. Numerous herbs have shown promise in reducing common symptoms like pain, exhaustion, nausea, and sleeplessness. These symptoms may have a significant effect on the patient's quality of life and the overall course of treatment. Herbs like rhodiola (Rhodiola rosea) and ashwagandha (Withania somnifera) can help fight cancer-related exhaustion and boost energy levels. Ginger (Zingiber officinale) and peppermint (Mentha piperita) have been demonstrated to alleviate nausea and vomiting caused by chemotherapy. Furthermore, anti-inflammatory herbs like Boswellia (Boswellia serrata) and turmeric (Curcuma longa) may help reduce pain and inflammation related to cancer and its treatments.

Additionally, by specifically targeting cancer cells and preventing the formation of tumors, several herbs have direct anti-cancer properties that may enhance traditional cancer treatments. Natural substances with anti-inflammatory and antioxidant effects, such as those found in green tea (Camellia sinensis), turmeric, and grapes (resveratrol), have been shown to inhibit the growth of cancer cells, cause apoptosis (programmed cell death), and suppress angiogenesis in tumors (the creation of new blood vessels to support tumor growth). Herbal medicines can complement an all-encompassing integrative treatment strategy, improving the efficacy of conventional therapies and lowering the risk of cancer recurrence, even if they are not commonly utilized as stand-alone cancer treatments.

Furthermore, herbal medicine provides patients and their families with emotional and spiritual support in addition to physical symptom management in integrative cancer therapy. Herbs with relaxing and mood-stabilizing qualities, such as chamomile (Matricaria chamomilla), lavender (Lavandula angustifolia), and lemon balm (Melissa officinalis), can help lower anxiety, encourage relaxation, and enhance the quality of sleep. Practitioners can address the psychological and emotional effects of cancer diagnosis and treatment by including these herbs in supportive care regimens. This helps patients and their loved ones feel resilient and well-being.

Furthermore, incorporating herbal medicine into integrative cancer care underscores the significance of customized treatment regimens based on the particular requirements, preferences, and situations of every patient. With the wide range of possibilities provided by herbal medicines, medical professionals can tailor treatment plans to the specific type, stage, and goals of the cancer and any other medical disorders. Through individualized care, professionals can address each patient's unique obstacles and worries, enabling them to participate actively in their recovery.

In conclusion, herbal medicine makes a substantial contribution to integrative cancer care by offering supportive care that considers the psychological, emotional, and spiritual dimensions of cancer in addition to a thorough therapeutic approach. Herbal medications have the potential to improve treatment results and the quality of life for cancer patients by enhancing immune function, managing side effects, counteracting the adverse effects of conventional therapy, and providing emotional support. To ensure safety, effectiveness, and compatibility with other treatments, patients receiving active cancer treatment must speak with a certified healthcare expert before beginning any herbal regimen. Incorporating herbal medicine with conventional cancer care can be beneficial. It offers patients complete support and improves their general well-being throughout the cancer journey with careful integration and tailored advice.

Addressing Chronic Pain with Herbal Remedies

Millions of individuals worldwide suffer from chronic pain, a widespread and crippling ailment that frequently reduces quality of life and makes daily tasks more difficult. While some people find relief from chronic pain through traditional therapies like medication and physical therapy, others may turn to alternative methods like herbal remedies. A natural and comprehensive approach to pain treatment is provided by herbal therapy, as many herbs include analgesic, anti-inflammatory, and muscle- relaxing qualities that can aid in pain relief and healing.

The most well-known herb for treating pain is turmeric (Curcuma longa), a vibrant yellow herb that can be found in Indian cuisine and traditional medicine. Curcumin, a bioactive substance found in turmeric, has been demonstrated to have potent analgesic and anti-inflammatory effects. Clinical research has shown that taking supplements containing turmeric can effectively reduce pain and inflammation in illnesses like fibromyalgia, rheumatoid arthritis, and osteoarthritis. Turmeric's antioxidant qualities also aid in preventing oxidative stress, which can worsen pain and cause tissue damage.

Another herb that has long been used to treat chronic pain is ginger (Zingiber officinale), which has potent analgesic and anti-inflammatory qualities. Gingerol and school, which are present in ginger, decrease the creation of inflammatory mediators and the perception of pain. Research has indicated that taking supplements containing ginger may be beneficial in treating conditions such as osteoarthritis, menstrual cramps, and migraine headaches. Research has indicated that taking supplements containing ginger may be beneficial in treating conditions such as osteoarthritis, menstrual cramps, and migraine headaches. Ginger has also long been used to manage the usual adverse effects of chronic pain drugs and therapies, such as nausea and vomiting.

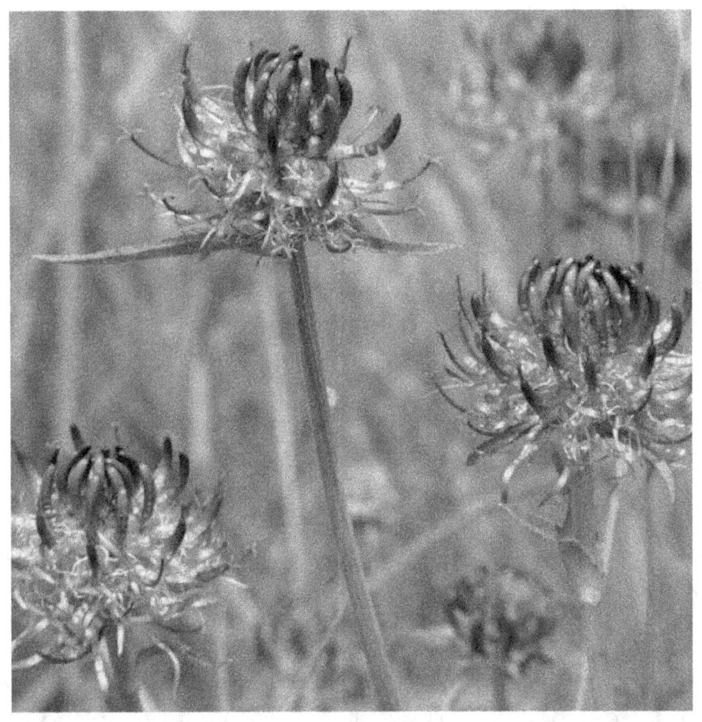

Furthermore, devil's Claw (Harpagophytum procumbens) and white willow bark (Salix alba) are two plants that have long been used by people as pain and inflammation relievers. Devil's Claw contains iridoid glycosides called harpagosides, which have been shown to have analgesic and anti-inflammatory properties as well as the ability to lessen osteoarthritis and low back pain symptoms. Comparably, salicin, a substance found in white willow bark, is converted into salicylic acid, which functions similarly to aspirin regarding analgesic and anti-inflammatory properties. With no chance of reliance or gastrointestinal adverse effects, these herbs offer natural alternatives to prescription painkillers.

Herbs with sedative and muscle-relaxing qualities, such as kava (Piper methysticum) and valerian (Valeriana officinalis), can also help relieve discomfort associated with stress and encourage relaxation. Valerian root contains valeric acid and valepotriates, which work on the central nervous system to cause relaxation and lessen muscle spasms. Similarly, kavalactones in kava have anxiolytic and muscle-relaxing properties that can relieve pain and encourage sound sleep. These herbs are beneficial for people who are dealing with chronic pain brought on by tension in their muscles, stress, or anxiety.

Furthermore, the use of herbal medicine in the treatment of chronic pain underscores the significance of attending to underlying imbalances and exacerbating factors of pain. Herbs like skullcap (Scutellaria lateriflora) and St. John's Wort (Hypericum perforatum) can enhance emotional well-being and lessen anxiety and sadness symptoms, frequently linked to chronic pain. Herbal remedies help patients build abilities to cope while addressing the emotional and mental components of pain in order to improve their general standard of life.

Moreover, combining dietary changes, physical activity, and stress reduction methods can improve the efficacy of herbal treatments for persistent pain. A well-rounded diet rich in anti-inflammatory foods such as fruits, whole grains, and omega-3 oils can help reduce pain and inflammation. Frequent physical activity can help increase flexibility, strength, and mobility while lowering the intensity of symptoms associated with chronic pain. This includes stretching, strength training, and low-impact activities like yoga and swimming. In addition, stress-reduction methods like progressive muscle relaxation, deep breathing, and meditation can support the benefits of herbal medicines by easing muscle tension and fostering calm.

To sum up, herbal medicine presents beneficial choices for managing persistent pain, offering organic substitutes for traditional therapies, and encouraging all-encompassing recovery. Herbs, including devil's Claw, valerian, turmeric, and ginger, have sedative, analgesic, and anti-inflammatory qualities that can help people with chronic pain disorders feel better and manage their pain better. Before starting any herbal regimen, you should see an experienced physician to ensure that it is safe and effective, especially if you are using a prescription or have a history of medical issues. Herbal medicines can be used with other holistic approaches and lifestyle improvements to help people manage their pain more effectively and improve their general health.

CHAPTER XIV

Herbal Medicine and Environmental Sustainability

Promoting Sustainable Cultivation and Harvesting Practices

The focus has shifted recently to herbal medicines as possible sources of antiviral components. Herbal medicine has long been popular due to its historical applications and ability to offer supplementary or alternative therapies to those found in mainstream medications. However, it is essential to support sustainable growing and harvesting methods to realize the full antiviral potential of these herbal remedies. Sustainable practices preserve biodiversity and the health of ecosystems while ensuring the longevity of populations of medicinal plants.

The implementation of organic agricultural practices is a crucial component of sustainable agriculture. The use of artificial fertilizers and pesticides, which can degrade soil quality and contaminate herbal products with dangerous residues, is avoided in organic farming. Herbal producers that adopt organic farming practices reduce their environmental impact and yield premium herbs devoid of chemical residues that may impair their medicinal properties. Furthermore, using organic farming techniques results in better ecosystems that encourage the growth of medicinal plants by increasing soil fertility and biodiversity.

Promoting agroforestry systems can improve the sustainability of herbal production and organic farming. Agroforestry improves biodiversity and imitates natural ecosystems by incorporating trees and bushes into agricultural landscapes. Farmers can produce microclimates that support plant growth and serve as a habitat for beneficial species by intercropping medicinal plants with trees. Agroforestry systems help farmers diversify their income streams and become less dependent on a particular crop by providing them with several revenue streams. In addition, trees reduce atmospheric carbon dioxide, reducing climate change's impacts and enhancing environmental resilience overall.

Ethical harvesting methods are an essential component of sustainable herbal cultivation. The over-harvesting of medicinal plants has the potential to reduce natural populations, endangering biodiversity and their long-term survival. Establishing harvesting quotas based on scientific evaluations of population dynamics and growth rates is crucial to preventing overexploitation. Promoting selective harvesting methods also guarantees that only mature plants are taken, allowing younger plants to increase and repopulate the area. Herbalists and wildcrafters can guarantee future generations' access to medicinal plants by implementing sustainable harvesting practices.

Moreover, sustainable herbal production is greatly aided by community-based conservation programs. Local communities gain a sense of guardianship and ownership over their natural resources when they are involved in conservation activities. To lessen the strain on wild plant species, community-led projects can create protected areas, put in place rotational harvesting plans, and offer substitute sources of income. By enabling local communities to responsibly manage their natural resources, we can increase resilience and ensure that the advantages of producing herbal medicines are distributed fairly.

In addition, certification programs like FairWild and organic certifications give customers peace of mind that herbal goods are supplied ethically. Customers can support sustainable herbal production techniques and help conserve biodiversity by selecting items certified under these schemes. Supporting ethical brands and small-scale herbal producers also helps to create a more robust and fair herbal medicine supply chain that is advantageous to both consumers and producers.

In conclusion, utilizing the antiviral properties of herbal medicine requires encouraging sustainable farming and harvesting methods. We can maintain the long-term viability of medicinal plant populations while preserving biodiversity and the health of ecosystems by embracing agroforestry systems, implementing responsible harvesting practices, encouraging community-based conservation projects, and adopting organic farming methods. By working together, we can fully utilize herbal medicine's abilities to treat viral infections while advancing social justice, environmental sustainability, and consumer choice. The focus has shifted recently to herbal medicines as possible sources of antiviral components.

Herbal medicine has long been popular due to its historical applications and ability to offer supplementary or alternative therapies to those found in mainstream medications. However, supporting sustainable growing and harvesting methods is essential to fully realizing these herbal remedies' antiviral potential. Sustainable practices preserve biodiversity and the health of ecosystems while ensuring the longevity of populations of medicinal plants.

The implementation of organic agricultural practices is a crucial component of sustainable agriculture. The use of artificial fertilizers and pesticides, which can degrade soil quality and contaminate herbal products with dangerous residues, is avoided in organic farming. Herbal producers that adopt organic farming practices reduce their environmental impact and yield premium herbs devoid of chemical residues that may impair their medicinal properties. Furthermore, using organic farming techniques results in better ecosystems that encourage the growth of medicinal plants by increasing soil fertility and biodiversity.

Promoting agroforestry systems can improve the sustainability of herbal production and organic farming. Agroforestry improves biodiversity and imitates natural ecosystems by incorporating trees and bushes into agricultural landscapes. Farmers can produce microclimates that support plant growth and serve as a habitat for beneficial species by intercropping medicinal plants with trees. Agroforestry systems help farmers diversify their income streams and become less dependent on a particular crop by providing them with several revenue streams. Likewise, trees collect carbon dioxide from the atmosphere, which lessens the consequences of climate change and improves environmental resilience in general.

Ethical harvesting methods are an essential component of sustainable herbal cultivation. The over-harvesting of medicinal plants has the potential to reduce natural populations, endangering biodiversity and their long-term survival. Establishing harvesting quotas based on scientific evaluations of population dynamics and growth rates is crucial to preventing overexploitation. Promoting selective harvesting methods also guarantees that only mature plants are taken, allowing younger plants to increase and repopulate the area. Herbalists and wildcrafters can guarantee future generations' access to medicinal plants by implementing sustainable harvesting practices.

Moreover, sustainable herbal production is greatly aided by community-based conservation programs. Local communities gain a sense of guardianship and ownership over their natural resources when they are involved in conservation activities. To lessen the strain on wild plant species, community-led projects can create protected areas, put in place rotational harvesting plans, and offer substitute sources of income. By enabling local communities to manage their natural resources responsibly, we can increase resilience and ensure that the advantages of producing herbal medicines are distributed fairly.

In addition, certification programs like FairWild and organic certifications give customers peace of mind that herbal goods are supplied ethically. Customers can support sustainable herbal production techniques and help conserve biodiversity by selecting items certified under these schemes. Supporting ethical brands and small-scale herbal producers also helps to create a more robust and fair herbal medicine supply chain that is advantageous to both consumers and producers.

In conclusion, utilizing the antiviral properties of herbal medicine requires encouraging sustainable farming and harvesting methods. We can maintain the long-term viability of medicinal plant populations while preserving biodiversity and the health of ecosystems by embracing agroforestry systems, implementing responsible harvesting practices, encouraging community-based conservation projects, and adopting organic farming methods. By working together, we can fully utilize herbal medicine's abilities to treat viral infections while advancing social justice, environmental sustainability, and consumer choice.

Conservation Efforts for Endangered Medicinal Plants

Numerous medicinal plants with intriguing antiviral effects can be found in our planet's incredible biodiversity. However, many species of medicinal plants are in danger of going extinct due to the unrelenting exploitation of natural resources, habitat damage, and climate change.

Coordination of conservation activities is essential to harness the antiviral properties of herbs while maintaining the sustainability of these resources.

Protecting and restoring habitat is a critical component in conserving endangered medicinal plants. Ensuring the survival of endangered plant species requires the restoration of degraded habitats and the preservation of intact ecosystems. A critical sanctuary for rare and imperiled medicinal plants, protected areas like national parks and nature reserves keep their ecosystems safe from encroachment and unsustainable exploitation. Furthermore, habitat restoration and forestry programs aid in reconstructing favorable conditions necessary for the regeneration and proliferation of endangered plants.

Ex-situ conservation efforts are essential for preserving endangered medicinal plants and habitat conservation. As living plant collections are housed and seeds are preserved for future generations, botanical gardens, arboreta, and seed banks function as genetic diversity repositories. These conservation centers provide insurance against the extinction of plant species in the wild, in addition to being living labs for study and teaching. Ex-situ conservation initiatives assist in keeping rare medicinal plants from becoming extinct by carefully cultivating and propagating them, which makes it easier for them to be reintroduced into restored ecosystems.

Moreover, neighborhood-based conservation programs enable nearby communities to take on the role of guardians for their natural resources. We can preserve medicinal plant species and their ecosystems by utilizing the traditional knowledge and wisdom of the indigenous peoples and local stakeholders involved in conservation initiatives. Indigenous groups frequently have solid cultural attachments to medicinal plants, and their customs can provide insightful information about managing habitats and sustainable harvesting methods.

By acknowledging and observing indigenous rights and customary knowledge systems, we advocate for culturally aware conservation strategies that uphold environmental sustainability and social justice.

Furthermore, policy frameworks and legal protection are necessary to prevent overexploitation and habitat damage of endangered medicinal plants. Passing laws governing medicinal plants' gathering, sale, and use discourages illicit harvesting and guarantees sustainable harvesting methods. Encouraging the recovery of endangered species and preventing overexploitation are two benefits of implementing quotas, licenses, and harvesting recommendations based on scientific assessments of the condition and trends of plant populations. Furthermore, encouraging global cooperation and collaboration in conservation initiatives can guarantee the preservation of migratory species and their habitats and improve the efficacy of conservation measures implemented across national boundaries.

Increasing public awareness of the value of protecting the biodiversity of medicinal plants is a crucial component of conservation initiatives. By emphasizing medicinal plants' ecological, cultural, and financial benefits, we encourage people to take action and protect these priceless resources on a personal and community level. Sustainable consumption habits, ethical sourcing, policy advocacy, education programs, outreach projects, and public engagement campaigns enable citizens to make educated decisions and support conservation efforts.

To sum up, conservation activities for endangered species are critical to sustainably harness the antiviral properties of these therapeutic plants. We can protect nature's pharmacy and guarantee the availability of medicinal plants for upcoming generations by integrating habitat conservation, ex-situ conservation, community-based methods, legal protection, and public education. By working together, we can preserve ecosystems, conserve biodiversity, and fully utilize herbal medicine's power to treat viral diseases while advancing social justice and environmental sustainability.

CONCLUSION

To provide a thorough guide for battling viral infections, "Tapping into Herbal Antiviral Powers: Blending Tradition and Science in Fighting Viruses" expertly unites the traditional knowledge of herbal medicine with contemporary scientific understanding. The book clarifies the effectiveness of herbal treatments in boosting the body's immune system and preventing viral infections through thorough study and perceptive analysis. By integrating cutting-edge scientific research with conventional wisdom, the writer offers readers a comprehensive strategy for preventing and treating viral infections.

The author frequently emphasizes the value of evidence-based procedures in the book to give readers the confidence to incorporate herbal treatments into their daily routines. The book also emphasizes the perennial effectiveness of nature's pharmacy in treating viral illnesses by examining the historical use of herbs in many cultures and civilizations.

The book's accessibility is among its best features. All readers can quickly grasp the content because complex scientific concepts are presented in an easily understood manner. Furthermore, valuable hints and recipes enable readers to utilize herbs' antiviral properties in everyday situations.

To summarize, "Tapping into Herbal Antiviral Powers" is a priceless tool for anyone looking to strengthen their immune system and fight viral infections organically. The book provides a road map for achieving optimal health and well-being in the face of viral dangers by fusing tradition and science. It requires reading for everybody interested in holistic approaches to well-being.

Thank you for buying and reading/ listening to our book. If you found this book useful/ helpful please take a few minutes and leave a review on the platform where you purchased our book. Your feedback matters greatly to us.